Rapid Cognitive Therapy

The Professional Therapist's Guide To Rapid Change Work
Volume 1

Georges Philips
and
Terence Watts

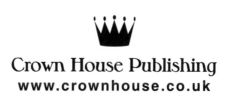

Crown House Publishing
www.crownhouse.co.uk

Published in the UK by

Crown House Publishing Limited
Crown Buildings
Bancyfelin
Carmarthen
Wales
SA33 5ND
UK
www.crownhouse.co.uk

First published 1999
Reprinted 2001, 2004

British Library of Cataloguing-in-Publication Data
A catalogue entry for this book is available from the British Library.

ISBN 1899836373

LCCN 2004108817

Printed and bound in the UK by
The Cromwell Press
Trowbridge
Wiltshire

Dedications

To my lovely Lyndy
whose faith is my oasis
with love always

Georges

To my wife, whose support
has forever remained constant

Terence

Table of Contents

Part Three: Non-analytical Work

Part Four: Tidying up

Part Five: Miscellaneous

Acknowledgements

We would like to thank
the following people for their advice and guidance
during the writing of this book ...

Dr. Chris Forester
Dr. Joe Keaney, Ireland
Vera Peiffer
Jacquelyne Morison
Penny Parks
Keith Beesley
Tony Jennings
Lyne Driscoll
John & Litsa Trikka
Prof V M Mathew
Dr David Pugh MB BS
Mehmet Adali

Preface

Welcome!

Congratulations. You have just bought one of the most important books that you will ever have on your bookshelf. Georges Philips and Terence Watts have pooled their considerable work experience and written a practical guide for brief therapy which goes way beyond the mere description of theoretical principles and the dry outline of methods and techniques. *Rapid Cognitive Therapy* is a course in enabling your clients to be successful in their endeavour to overcome not just their presenting problems but also all the other problems that they never got round to telling you about.

Even though Philips and Watts are hypnotherapists and psychotherapists, their methodology is still relevant and can be used with slight modification for many other types of therapy such as NLP, Gestalt, behaviourist and analytical approaches. Not only will you find lucid explanations of how beliefs come about and how we are subconsciously influenced by our personality on the one hand and by our environment and experiences on the other, but you are also presented with structures for the first few sessions as well as full scripts for analytical and non-analytical work with the client.

Philips and Watts also give a lot of attention to client resistance, a problem which can easily sabotage an otherwise well-conducted session, as anyone will know who has been working as a therapist for any length of time. The way the authors resolve potential or actual resistance is not only very elegant but also highly effective, as you will find out when you use these methods in your own practice.

However, my main reason for recommending *Rapid Cognitive Therapy* to you is that it is an approach which is entirely respectful towards the client's fears and anxieties he or she brings into therapy. Philips and Watts approach has integrity and helps the client to actively confront difficult issues in a safe way so that the client can be successful in removing the stumbling blocks that are obstructing personal development.

The only thing that is better than reading this book is to go and see Philips and Watts in action. If you want to learn effective ways to produce outstanding results that last, book yourself on to one of their courses or workshops and make sure you experience them live! You'll laugh a lot and you'll learn a lot, even if you are an experienced therapist. I know—I did.

Vera Peiffer
BA (Psychology)
Author of *Positive Thinking*

Foreword

We are living in a period when everyone is impatient and expects rapid response and change. The capacity for change—either positive or negative—lies within each individual. Every one of us is born with the ability to bring about whatever changes we need in order to cope with adverse situations. However, it is becoming increasingly obvious that individuals are finding it difficult to deal with the adversities of day-to-day life and are declaring: "I can't cope." The inability to cope with life in general—which I call 'acopia'—is a feature of modern society that will soon find its place in the English dictionary.

Life is simple. If one chooses to make it complicated, then one is entirely responsible for that choice. Indeed, there are times when one becomes so associated with a particular situation or problem that one is unable to be objective and becomes 'stuck' in negativity. It is the individual alone who can choose between being negative and being positive; as it is said: "Some are wise, some are otherwise."

In any therapy, the therapist should act only as a catalyst, facilitating the process of change or transformation while at the same time remaining unchanged or unaffected by the therapy. As a catalyst, the therapist should neither try to take credit for improvements nor accept blame for unresolved problems.

In the current atmosphere of rapid advances in technology, people are looking for immediate results, and long-winded, open-ended therapy is not acceptable to anyone other than those who wish to perpetuate their problems due to secondary gain. It is said that the neurotics come for therapy to perfect their neurosis. With increasing demands put on the caring professions and the disparity between supply and demand, it is not surprising that modern society is increasingly seeking new methods that are time-saving and cost-effective. There may be literally hundreds of approaches one can take to bring about positive change in the patient. Whatever method one uses, throughout treatment, the therapist's task is to guide the patient in an empathic and responsive manner to reach the established goals.

Rapid Cognitive Therapy provides a new psychotherapeutic approach whereby effective and positive changes can be brought about within a very short period. All the techniques described in this book can be used along with behavioural, analytical, and other modes of therapies. As well as describing the art of rapid cognitive therapy, the authors have provided therapists with the means to get started rapidly by outlining structures for the initial sessions as well as full scripts for analytical and non-analytical work with the client.

I am delighted to write the Foreword to *Rapid Cognitive Therapy*, written by two excellent and experienced therapists, to join the ranks of modern publications in the domain of psychotherapeutic approaches.

Professor VM Mathew
Consultant Psychiatrist
President: British Medical Hypnotherapy Examination Board

Introduction

The purpose of this book is to provide you, the therapist, with a powerful toolbox that will ensure that you are equipped to deal easily and effectively with the vast majority of psychological difficulties presented by your clients.

Every therapist has his own favoured methodology, along with a few reliable 'tricks of the trade' to help clients to get from where they are to where they want to be. Every therapist is also aware that he can never have access to too many 'tricks' or too many resources to help create change for his clients! The authors of this book each have many years of experience as professional 'hands-on' hypnotherapists and hypnoanalysts, and what is presented here is a distillation of their favourite techniques. It represents just a part of the unique therapeutic process that they have named *Rapid Cognitive Therapy*—RCT—which seamlessly marries cognitive work, visualisation, NLP, regression and analytical methods.

Rapid Cognitive Therapy

RCT is a client-centred, multi-faceted brief therapy that allows the rapid and effective resolution of all manner of psychological and emotional conflicts. This book includes in-depth coverage of the branch of RCT known as Rapid Cognitive Analysis. The name of the therapy is derived as follows:

RAPID—the intent is to resolve problems in the quickest time possible.

COGNITIVE—it does not rely on your client's accepting 'in good faith' a mysterious, half-understood mental process; instead, it allows him a full **understanding** *at the beginning of therapy* as to why he is the way he is. It does not leave a client wondering/worrying about how he will find that elusive 'forgotten traumatic event' nor, indeed, how he will search for anything that he does not already consciously know. It does not leave an individual fearful of what he might find or anxious about false memory, or somebody 'meddling with his mind'. Because of this, resistance is minimal, right from the beginning. During the analytical work, your client's increasing understanding of what ails him, and why, will inspire positive changes to his belief system, and allow him to assimilate those changes into his personality, which is the 'bottom-line' aim of most therapies.

THERAPY—it is a truly therapeutic process, working with the subconscious/preconscious part of the psyche, locating, analysing and thereby resolving active conflict(s) into acceptance.

Standard or traditional analytical (or 'regression-to-cause') therapies rely upon repression release, abreaction and catharsis to produce an alleviation of symptoms. While this is undoubtedly effective where a repressed traumatic emotional state is the root cause of an individual's difficulties, it has many shortcomings. It works best for hysterical illness—indeed it was for this sort of condition that the 'father' of analytical techniques, Sigmund Freud, invented free association. But not all our clients are suffering from a hysterical illness and while analysis and free associative techniques can help most psychological ills, there are undoubtedly better ways, faster and more effective methods, to help deal with a lot of the difficulties that the modern individual encounters in life.

With RCT, repression(s) will still be released and resolved via abreactive work when necessary, just as effectively, just as quickly—maybe even more so—as with standard analytical techniques. In addition, 'cumulative trauma' will be easily dealt with, too, while the process is still just as effective for the hysterical type of illness for which straightforward free association was developed.

One of the mainstay areas of therapeutic work lies in effectively resolving past hurts and unfinished subconscious 'business'. Because of this, the section on working with analysis and/or regression is fairly comprehensive, though this book is not intended as a full training course for these methodologies. If you have never used either methodology in a therapeutic session, though, there is more than enough here to get you safely started and whet your appetite to learn more. Although you can easily utilise a lot of RCT work successfully without employing either of these techniques, there will be many occasions when, using them, you will do far better things for your client.

With RCT, you can often be effective even working without hypnosis if necessary. You can also work easily with logical/analytically-minded clients and deal with relationship problems more effectively. You can resolve many difficulties in only one to three sessions and can often completely remove a 'social phobia' in only one session. In addition, it is easier to improve motivation or personal confidence, deal with unresolved grief issues and many more of the emotional ills that beset your clients.*

Because of the 'instantly available' culture of our modern society, there is a growing requirement and expectation among the public that we should be able to provide an expert and immediately available 'cure' for whatever problem they present us with. Not only that, the ever-increasing belief that life should be fun—and that it *is* fun for everybody else—means that the problems clients are bringing to us are becoming more wide-ranging than ever before. It is the therapist who can come closest to those client expectations who is destined to remain successful, far into the future!

RCT is probably the most complete therapeutic system available— an integrated, streamlined, matching 'set of tools' for all therapists. When you learn how to use RCT, you will be astonished at the way you suddenly become more effective, almost overnight!

*Not every technique that can be used with RCT is necessarily shown in this book, which is the first book on the subject.

Part One

Pre-Therapy

Chapter 1

Three Considerations

Whilst not particularly concerned with techniques, this chapter will be of help to all therapists in understanding the processes of memory and belief, as well as in recognising two important psychological situations which are capable of rendering even the best therapy useless in the long term unless they are properly addressed.

Memory and belief

Imagine, as vividly as you can, a trio of skinhead-type hooligans standing on a street corner, lager tins in hand, tattooed knuckles, DM boots—the lot. A middle-aged man comes out from a door opposite, carrying a briefcase, and one of the skinheads suddenly yells something before launching himself across the road, hurling himself at the man and wrestling him to the ground, grabbing at his briefcase.

What might you believe you have just observed? A mugging, maybe? That is the most obvious answer, after all. Or perhaps the skinhead lived in that house; it was his briefcase, and the man was a burglar. Perhaps, even, the skinhead was a plain-clothes detective and the man was someone the police have been after for months. Or maybe a film was being made. It could even be that it was nothing more than a boisterous joke and the man was his father—or his lover!

The facts of the scenario were always the same—but the interpretations are vastly different, depending greatly on your own individual thought process. Every memory you have is like that. It is the result of perception, pre-conception, beliefs, knowledge, interpretation and re-interpretation, all based very loosely on or around *fact*. It is an extremely unreliable mix and the bad news is that it is the best bit of what our clients bring with them to the consulting room as their contribution to therapy.

The good news is that if we understand certain concepts we can be more effective and therefore help people more easily. The understanding of the memory process is an important tool for a therapist and perhaps the most important understanding of all is this:

> *We act upon what we believe to be true, and we believe to be true what we think we remember.*

Since we act upon it, it helps to shape our personality and behaviour patterns and our expectation and belief systems. It matters not one jot that the belief may be patently ridiculous as far as the rest of the world is concerned. Our conscious critical faculty insists that what we know is so—unless and until we discover for ourselves that we were wrong in that belief, when we then have enlightenment and can begin to accommodate a change into our way of being.

The sky is green

This insistency of the conscious critical faculty is easy to illustrate. Imagine that somebody is trying to convince you that the sky is green and that grass is blue… of course, you would simply deny that this was the case and you would *know beyond doubt* that you were right. It is a belief upon which you act and the critical conscious faculty ensures that it remains so. But there will have been many times in your life when you have been just as convinced of 'the truth', just as certain of your facts, just as sure that you were right, only to discover that you were, in fact, wrong.

That is just how it is for your clients. They are all harbouring a belief upon which they are acting, yet which is based upon false perception, even though that false perception may not necessarily be responsible for their symptoms. But here is something very important: if a client believes, say, that she has been abducted by aliens, *truly believes it to the point where she 'knows' it happened*, then that belief will be accommodated into her behaviour and expectation system just as surely as if it *were* true. It will affect the client *just as surely as if it **were** true*. The same goes for anything the client believes, no matter how unlikely, how outrageous, how bizarre. It is the client's truth and that is what we must work with, and though we work with that 'truth' via her memory, it is belief, not memory, that holds the key to her neuroses.

Memory is not detailed

Before progressing further with the implications of all this as far as therapy is concerned, we will have a quick look at one or two aspects of the way that memory works.

Memory is not generally very detailed. If you remember a day out at a pleasure park, for example, what you will actually remember is that you went there, along with the recall of a few 'stills', as it were, from your visit, rather than remembering the whole visit from beginning to end. If you remember a visit to a shop, how much detail could you recall about the other customers? Or the colour of the till? Or the type of wristwatch the assistant was wearing? You can study a 'still' frame in your mind's eye for some time and not be certain, and it is that vagueness which gives us all sorts of problems, because, often, logic comes into play to fill in the gaps without our ever knowing that this has happened. And the gaps are filled by accessing other situations, concepts or experiences which are viewed as similar by the subconscious processes—similar, but very definitely part *of a **different** situation, concept or experience.* It is just about the nearest thing you will ever find to a genuine 'false memory', but like every other 'false memory', it is nothing more than a false belief—a different animal altogether.

Templates

The mind works on a series of templates—in this context, templates are images that have become familiar to us—that we have stored away in a sort of memory archive. We identify things and experiences by reference to these templates and it is when something does not properly 'fit' any of those that already exist, that a new one is formed—and instantaneously becomes part of our belief system. But what if the circumstance is so totally different from anything else we have experienced at any time in our life that we simply cannot identify it or any part of it? We would have no partial matches to go by and would need an explanation of what was happening before we could even begin to understand it. But because we had no pre-existing template to confirm our experience by, that explanation would not engender so strong a belief pattern as otherwise; we know that explanations are sometimes incorrect, so we would leave doubt 'in the frame'.

And here is something of enormous importance: templates are formed for *everything* we experience, whether it is reality or fantasy, whether it is fact or fiction. Now, to return to those individuals who are absolutely certain that they have been abducted by aliens—how did they come to develop that belief? Even assuming that the event really occurred, it is unlikely that an alien would explain to them they had been abducted by aliens. So they would need a template that was *similar* in order for them to recognise their 'truth', and that template can only have come from a fictional or 'hearsay 'scenario. But when an individual appears to experience for herself something that is a match for even only a fictional template, then it becomes an absolute reality as far as she is concerned. She would have not a single shred of doubt and even the most sophisticated of lie detectors would indicate that she was telling the truth about what had happened, because she would, indeed, be telling the 'truth' *as far as she was concerned*. More importantly, she may very well fear that such an abduction might happen again and develop an entire set of symptoms designed specifically to avoid such a likelihood. Agoraphobia, of course, is a distinct possibility—the result of the mind acting upon a belief.

That is what a client's truth is. As far as she is concerned, it is *the* truth.

Removing the stress

As far as therapy is concerned, it matters not at all whether what the client tells us is actually so; it is what she feels about it that counts, and we should treat it as if *were* fact and assist her in removing the stress from the situation. Only then can we do our job properly and help the client to find relief from her symptoms. Interestingly, even if you managed to persuade your client to *consciously* accept that what she had believed was not so, it is likely that she would still maintain her symptoms and may even feel worse, since there would now be no rationale. This is easy to test. Think of a person from your past whom you have always disliked—maybe a school teacher from your young years, a boss you never saw eye-to-eye with, or a family member who simply 'rubs you up the wrong way'. Now, imagine that it has been proven beyond doubt to you that this person is actually very respected and well-liked. Does that feel better? More likely, it hits resistance! Change would only come from within you, from your own understanding, not from that of others.

These erroneous beliefs may reside purely in the unconscious, based around events which appeared to happen many years ago and which have long since been lost to consciousness, though still being part of the fundamental belief-set of the individual. Then, of course, there can be a quite dramatic shift during hypnoanalysis when an adult's understanding is brought to bear upon a situation which may have been almost incomprehensible to a child.

To put the point of this section in a nutshell: if your client believes something which you are certain is not true, let her carry on believing it, if you do not want to run the risk of creating a resistant state. Simply work on the resultant emotional states and let her find her own way to the truth if she wants to.

Cumulative Trauma

Cumulative Trauma, as its name implies, is created by a 'chain' of apparently minor events, any one of which would not be severe enough on its own to cause a problem. Taken as a whole, though, the effects can be profound and can cause severe neurosis. You can think of it as sixteen separate ounces of trauma as compared to a single solid pound of repression.

The major difference between trauma caused by a single event and cumulative trauma is that, most of the time, the events in a cumulative trauma pattern have not been repressed. They may still be 'invisible' though, because they seem absolutely 'normal'. The *events* may not have been repressed—but the *emotion* certainly has, and the individual's self-imagery and belief systems are inevitably affected. The sufferer from this condition will often describe her childhood as uncomfortable or awkward.

Cumulative Trauma may arise in at least two different ways:

(1) The constant repetition of a negative idea or circumstances over a long period of time, probably years. This continuous programming of a suggestible child carries on to the point where the child simply ceases to listen consciously. And that's when the damage is done, because the subconscious definitely does *not* stop listening and takes these suggestions 'on board' quite readily. It can also be brought about by continual ridicule, rejection, dismissal of achievement, or perceived humiliation. It is convenient to think of this as Simple Cumulative Trauma.

(2) Fate ensuring the repetition of like events that threaten the life requirements—security and survival—of the child. For instance, Mother leaves, Father finds life impossible and hands the child to other relatives; they can't cope and send the child into care; the foster or adoptive family breaks up; bullying at school, the first firm that she works for goes bust... Then the urge to repeat takes over, emotional relationships start to founder... and so the whole process goes on. This creates Compound Cumulative Trauma.

You should find out about the sort of events at (2) during the initial interview and fact-gathering session. You can be in for quite a job with an individual who has suffered compound cumulative trauma, because getting her to reframe her life events and revise her opinion of herself is not going to be easy.

The individual with simple cumulative trauma is easier to help, though you could easily miss her problems for a very simple reason—it is so much a part of your client's normal life routine that she simply doesn't bother to tell you about it. It may even be that she has forgotten about it temporarily. Not repressed, though. We've had many a client say something like: "Oh, yes, that's right, I'd forgotten about that. He was always telling me I was (thick... or stupid... fat... clumsy... idiotic... a wimp... etc.)." Sometimes it has been just a continual harangue of general ineffectiveness, worthlessness and/or uselessness.

There will often be a pause after a client has remembered something of that nature. If she ventures no further down that path, we might say, quite casually: "I wonder what other people might think about an adult who constantly drums it into a child that she's..." It might take a few moments for the 'penny to drop' but when it does, we have a route into the very core of our client's problem(s).

It all comes down to expectation and belief. The child was brain-washed to the point where she does not realise that there is anything amiss with her thought processes. After all, it was taught and insisted upon—it has become an automatic (and therefore hidden) thinking pattern, a conditioned response entirely normal to the client. So she actually *knows* she is irretrievably stupid or clumsy or fat, or whatever has been programmed into her—it is a type of self-fulfilling prophesy. And if it is expected and believed, the subconscious will make certain that it continues to exist, via continual negative self-programming.

It can be more subtle. An anorexic individual may have been told as a fat child (and many anorexics have been fat children): "Nobody ever loves a fatty." The obese individual may have been taught that if she doesn't eat up all her food, she is of less value as a person. ("There are lots of children who would think themselves lucky...")

The symptoms can also be reversed. The fat child/adult eats for comfort because she is fat and therefore unlovable. And the thin child who becomes an anorexic adult tries not to eat at all because her parents' concerned reaction to her thinness and low appetite has created an association of anxiety with eating.

Unfortunately, there is no easy way to unravel the thinking processes that have been created by compound cumulative trauma. If there were, we could probably cure it by a simple suggestion. After all, the idea was put there by a suggestion in the first place, so a powerful enough counter-suggestion should deal with it. In fact, the respected American therapist, Michael Yapko, in his book *Trancework*, expresses the opinion that indirect suggestion will allow the mind to resolve its difficulties and conflicts without the creation of any substitute symptoms. Experience has shown that this is, indeed, quite often the case.

But not always. The subconscious, unreasoning and unthinking and only 'understanding' the need to discharge urges and drives, will sometimes produce a substitute anxiety expression. These new symptoms may well not be evident until a few months have passed, when the client may well not recognise that she is still suffering from the same psychological problem. Symptom substitution can be repeated a great many times, and each time there is a substitution it tends to become wider-based in the psyche, creating ever-growing problems.

Another problem is that we can never know beyond doubt that we are dealing with some form of cumulative trauma. And, of course, if the presenting problem had been caused not by this but by repression of an event in earlier years, then the emotion associated with that event must be released from repression to ensure continuing good emotional health in the client.

The answer here lies in some other form of regression-to-cause therapy. But you need to have your wits about you to spot that you are, in fact, dealing with cumulative trauma. If you do not, and you fail to subtly draw your client's attention to her 'hidden' thinking process in some way, you could spend an awful long time waiting for that elusive repression to surface. Much of the time, it is actually not a repression release that's needed; it is a fresh understanding of something that has been kicking around the (almost) conscious mind for years.

By far the most common symptom with this sort of trauma is low confidence and poor self-esteem. Of course, it is not fair to say that these symptoms are *always* caused by cumulative trauma, neither should it be assumed that those symptoms are always present. But they are good pointers.

Some other indicators are when your client continually apologises or repeatedly says things like:

"I'm sorry, I'm a bit slow sometimes."

"I'm just a bit stupid, I suppose."

"I'm not actually very bright."

"I know other people are a lot worse off than me."

"It was just the same when I was at school."

"I know it sounds silly, but..."

"I'm sorry to be such a nuisance."

Self-denigrating statements of this type—and there are very many more—have been *learnt* from somebody or via some thought process; they are not simply the product of self-evaluation.

It is when therapy—especially analytical therapy—is under way that we find our biggest clue to whether we are dealing with repression or with cumulative trauma. The client who presents with problems that have started suddenly as an adult and worsened rapidly, is probably being affected by a repression which has been triggered. Those who come to us claiming that they have had their symptom pattern since they were children are actually more likely to be suffering from some form of **conditioned response pattern**—the effect of cumulative trauma. In these cases, there will usually be a fair amount of emotional work right from the start.

The most important thing with cumulative trauma is to get to the underlying *idea* that has been instilled/taught and work on that. Simply overriding the symptom(s) with suggestion will work, but with a limited 'shelf life', because the belief system will not have been touched at all.

Hypervigilance

We all get clients 'suffering' from this condition in our consulting rooms, but it is rare indeed for it to be given as a presenting symptom. Put simply, it is a condition where the individual concerned holds an inner belief that she has to be totally on her guard every waking moment of every day, wherever she is and whatever she is doing.

It can lead to all sorts of obsessive behaviour patterns as well as producing difficulties with social interaction, relationship problems, and paranoid thought processes. It can cause problems 'on the couch', because there will be a tendency not to relax as much as we would like and almost certainly some difficulty in entering even a light state of trance. It is essential that we recognise and deal effectively with it, since trying to conduct a satisfactory session of either suggestive or analytic therapy without doing so is likely to be at best frustrating, at worst, a complete waste of time. Some therapists automatically diagnose it and conduct their session accordingly, almost without being aware that they are doing so but for those less experienced, a few pointers may help.

The hypervigilant individual has learned, at some point, that it is desirable to be very wary at all times, so wary that absolutely nothing escapes her attention. It can be caused by a single repressed memory, especially if the individual swore at the time that she would *never ever* allow anything like it to happen to them again, but the most likely cause is some form of Cumulative Trauma.

Whatever the origins of the problem, the hypervigilant individual will never drop her guard, even for an instant, in the normal way, and views being relaxed as an extremely vulnerable situation. That feeling is only partly in the conscious mind, and at a subconscious level is certainly linked to the 'fight or flight' response and therefore to mortality and survival. What she is looking out for, even though she is not consciously aware of the fact, is evidence that what she subconsciously fears is about to attack her; it does not matter that we know she is safe in our consulting room—her subconscious does not understand that concept, so she does not.

Needless to say, we have to do something about that if our efforts are to be of any use. We will come to that later on, but first, a few more symptoms of hyperviligance and then some questions we can ask to reveal its presence.

Among the indicators of this syndrome are: a dislike of the suggestion to close the eyes; an uneasiness about being in front of the therapist in the first place; evasiveness when answering questions of a personal nature; poor sleep patterns; excessive justification of presenting symptoms; instant, categorical dismissal of the idea that her reasons for her symptoms may be an erroneous association; a tendency to answer questions indirectly—often with another question. Mostly, she tends to be predominantly an RO personality (see Chapter Three) but hypervigilance is certainly not unknown in other personality groups. There will always be an RO influence, though.

Questions to ask

Each 'Yes' response to the first five questions is an indicator of the hypervigilant personality, as is each 'No' response to questions 6–10:

(1)   Do you tend to wake up more than once during the night?

(2)   Do you tend to have trouble getting to sleep in the first place?

(3)   Do you tend to feel uncomfortable in crowded places?

(4)   Do you find yourself truly disliking people for no reason?

(5)   Do you feel uncomfortable if there are people standing behind you—in a queue, perhaps?

(6)   Could you easily fall asleep in public—in a crowded train carriage, for example?

(7)   Is it possible for people to fool you, to 'pull the wool over your eyes'?

(8)   Do you feel at ease with strangers?

(9)   Do you find it easy to trust people once you know them?

(10) Can you 'let your hair down' easily at parties, or on occasions when other people are doing so?

Five or more 'correct' answers out of those ten questions, along with a few of the other indicators, means it is pretty certain that your client has a degree of hypervigilance that needs proper handling; more than that suggests that you will have difficulty getting this individual through satisfactory therapy, if at all.

Method

Getting her to relax is unlikely; the best we can manage is to get her focused, get the psyche turned inwards for once. The best form of induction is one that there can be no arguing with—if you suggest relaxation, she can argue afterwards that she was *not* relaxed at all, so she clearly didn't 'go under'. Attempts at using imagery will often produce: "But I just can't see that star (or stairs or whatever)..." or something similar. Any attempts at trance ratification, especially with any form of eyelock (just try telling someone who believes that she must be constantly on guard that her eyes are 'stuck tight, tight, shut'!), are almost certainly doomed to failure. So it is useful to employ an almost 'non-refusable' induction, along the lines of:

> "...now I want you to be aware of how your body is in the chair as you just lie there... being aware of the position of your arms, your legs... noticing, perhaps the weight of your head as it rests against the back of the chair... maybe feeling the texture of the arms of the chair against the palms of your hands, perhaps noticing whether there seems to be more weight in one arm than the other... or one leg or the other... or perhaps just being aware that your body is exactly as you want it to be... familiar, safe feelings... so that you can feel... just comfortable within yourself..." etc.

In other words, nothing that can be challenged or disputed, but everything that will lead to concentration upon *self*, with the 'natural' use of such words as *familiar, safe, comfortable*, and so on. It is also useful to *"wonder if you can use the power of your mind to control your heartbeat... just to slow that heartbeat down, just a little..."* etc.

You might find a hypnotic flush occurring and you might not; if you use a bio-feedback device, you may find the reading changing, but then again, you might not. So you will have to use your judgement as to when it is the right time to start whatever work you have decided to do with this client. But whenever that is, you will need to weave into the end of that induction some item from the client's history as she has reported it to you during your information-gathering, to get her mind and concentration where you need it to be. It could be seen as 'leading', but it is stuff that she has told you before and that therefore has a place in her psyche. And besides, if you do not do that she will be likely to flip back into guard mode and start analysing what has happened to and around her while she has lain on your couch.

If you are working with any form of causal event therapy—hypno-analysis or regression—there will almost always be one thing the client tells you, at some point, that should obviously have more emotion attached than there seems to be or to have been; save this until the right moment. That moment is when *she* mentions it again, during a session, usually with some sign of mild unease. Then… go for it! Hit her with every trick you know that will get her to release the emotion: repeat the image back to her, with feeling; ask her where in the body she *felt* that event; ask where she is feeling it now; if she denies it, ask her to imagine how it would feel and where she would feel it if she *were* feeling it right now; anything you can think of. You *might* be wrong, of course. This might be the wrong event… but the emotional work being suggested will often be enough to place her exactly where she should be. In any case, it is the best you are likely to be able to do with this sort of character and you are going to come a lot closer to success than you ever would with more relaxed or permissive methods.

Chapter 2

Making Change Desirable

Although your client wants relief from his presenting condition, he does not necessarily want to change. He knows he does not like the way he is or the way 'things' are, but there is very often a subconscious anxiety about a future that is unknown to him. He cannot know how he will be when he is not as he is—and it scares him. Quite often, in fact, he presents himself for therapy because he *wants* to change something about his life, but he just cannot seem to *do* it, no matter how hard he tries.

There are many times when an individual will 'hang on' to a situation in the hope that it will somehow improve, long after it has become obvious to everybody else in the world that there is little or no chance of this. This is especially true of relationships, though it can easily manifest itself in a great many other areas of life. Usually, the client will be blaming himself for the difficulty—he will feel that it is all his fault and will often present himself to you to get 'sorted out'. Well, sometimes we discover that he is right, when we go about the business of sorting him out… but more often than not, resistance is at work and it is very apparent that it is the problem which is the problem!

The reason for resistance to change of any sort is simple and linked closely to the survival complex: *if whatever you have been doing for x number of years has resulted in survival* (and it has, because you are still here!) *then you had better keep on doing it to **continue** to survive.* This will never be a conscious process; that will be far more logically presented and will involve lack of money, inability to cope, moral indebtedness, inadequacy, loyalty, or any one of a whole host of other reasons.

So we have to have the tools available to create not just a *willingness* for change to take place, but a genuine *desire* for it to do so, come what may, if we are to be effective for our clients.

Buttons

This particular method of facilitating a desire for change is especially effective, due to its interactive nature; the client has to actually *do* something, rather than simply employ thought. Realisation is quickly achieved, and because it is combined with a positive motor action, it is far more powerful than it might be otherwise.

The way the process is introduced to the client is important. The following, or something like it, works well:

> *"I'd like to explain something to you about one of the ways that the subconscious works, because it really is a remarkable part of our mind. What is often not realised is that, once it has initiated a course of action, it will not rest until it has somehow achieved what it has set out to do… And it really will do the most amazing and scarcely believable things to get to where it wants to go.*
>
> *"It will change your body language, the things you say, the way you think, the way you feel—physically as well as mentally. It will even cause your body chemistry to change the way you actually smell, if it sees that as a way to complete the plan. And it will have its way, make no mistake about it!*
>
> *"Now, the subconscious won't initiate any course of action, except under the right circumstances. There are two main reasons it might do so. One is when it believes it's necessary, even if you don't, and the other is when it believes that you want that course of action whole-heartedly. That's why positive thinking works—we set our sights well and truly on a goal and the subconscious does everything it can to help us reach it. It doesn't actually take a huge event to start that process in motion, actually, just a simple thought or an action, or better still, a thought and an action combined. Now, I believe we can easily get your subconscious mind to start working today for your benefit… we're going to combine a thought and an action to get it started. Does that seem like a good idea to you?"*

There are very few clients who will disagree with this, though it can happen, and then you are actually in a good position. He is probably already aware of what is inhibiting him and it is there to be worked at. In the normal way, however, you will get agreement, when you continue:

> *"Good, well done. Right, I want you to imagine that there is a button on each arm* (or side) *of your chair. Now, the left-hand button, if you press it, guarantees that **everything** in your life will stay just as it is... It'll get no worse, but then again, it'll get no better. That means that you will have... oh... what d'you think* (mention an appropriate number) *years more of it?* (Same number) *more years of exactly what you've got now. Maybe more... how would that feel?"*

Wait to see signs of a negative reaction from your client; if none appear, then draw his attention to the specific situations he has 'complained' about. Then:

> *"Now, the other button, the one at your right hand, guarantees change, guarantees that you will not have to put up with your situation for any longer than is necessary... Now, the big question..."*

Pause just long enough before you ask your client if he will push the left-hand button, the one that will keep him exactly as he is. Do this almost theatrically; lean slightly towards him and lower your voice a touch, adding:

> *"Will you...? Will you do that? Will you push that button and simply settle for what you've got, everything staying just the same... Remember, that subconscious of yours will obey what it thinks you really want... a thought and an action combined... Or do you really want to press the other button now, the one to make something happen? What do you think?"*

By far the vast majority of your clients will go for the change button. ***Now make him do it!*** Get him to actually press the imaginary change button—he will probably be in hypnosis by now if you've done your job properly and he will not think this at all unusual. The motor action involves your client in the quest for change and he will usually now readily accept that he actually *wants* change and that it will be good for him. It is a fairly safe assumption that resistance is now going to be less of a problem than it would otherwise have been.

Very few people will push the 'stay as you are' button; those that do are simply not ready to commit themselves to the idea of change and there is a need to work at this before therapy can progress successfully. They are truly not yet ready for therapy, though if you decide to seek to resolve their 'stuckness', a good starting point is: *"Tell me what you want to happen as a result of therapy."*

Catalysts

Sometimes, an individual simply cannot choose either course of action. He cannot contemplate staying as he is, but somewhere along the line there is fear about a possible aspect of change that he has consciously or unconsciously perceived but not addressed. This is where we need to discover whether it is something he cannot bear the idea of losing, or something that he is frightened of discovering or experiencing.

Here are a few useful catalytic interventions that can help to bring about a realisation within your client. They are orientated towards relationship issues, though they can easily be adapted to be useful in many other situations. The idea behind them is to bring a different perspective to the problem, from where change may be more accessible. In all cases, the 'follow-up' can follow normal therapeutic rules and needs no explanation here.

*"Are you anxious about losing what was **actually there**… or what you **hoped it would be**?"* Many people hang on to a relationship for this reason. In truth, it probably never has fulfilled their expectations but they have time and effort invested in it and are reluctant to admit their poor judgement and/or the 'wasted' months/years.

"Tell me how you helped this to happen, even if you didn't know at the time that that was what you were doing." Often, a client has had no awareness of this until the moment you ask him and you may have to help him probe. There usually is something. People introduce their partners to best friends; push them into joining a club or gym or similar; take up a time-consuming hobby; ignore warning signs like depression, non-responsiveness or staying at work late, etc. The client needs to find how he has contributed, because his resistance to change can be born out of the wish **not** to

confront his own part in the problem, even where his behaviour was completely innocent, maybe even supportive. Especially then, perhaps. A relationship breaking up is bad enough; for your client to have to recognise that it happened because of a voluntary behaviour on his part is even more painful. Follow up with: *"What did you want to happen when you did that?"* for more self-discovery, which often leads to the admission of 'mind games' that have backfired. When it does, you are home and dry: *"And what was it that made you decide to play that game…?"* This will highlight the true nature of the problem though you will probably need to pursue these last two questions with some tenacity!

"Tell me just one thing, **but only ONE thing,** *that you would choose to change about the way things are right now."* This can have the effect of focusing your client on the **real** nature of the problem. A good follow-up is: *"Now tell me how your life would be if that thing were changed."* Or something similar.

"That change button we talked about… what would have to happen before you could press it?" Self-explanatory.

"That 'stay as you are' button … what would have to happen before you could press that? How would you have to change? How would s/he have to change?" This carries a hidden suggestion to accept change, but it is more than that. Sometimes, *sometimes*, there is a simple solution to your client's difficulties, one that he has perceived as impossible to achieve. This will highlight it, and often you will be able to help him achieve it.

"What does s/he feel about all this?" Get your client's views, then: *"What do you think about his/her feelings?"* A focusing device which allows you to discover material to help with the change of state.

"Tell me how you will be and what you will be doing on the (give a date exactly one year away) *if nothing changes. Describe how your life will be then."* Do not accept "the same as it is now". Extract from your client as complete a description of a full day as possible. Follow with: *"And what would you* **like** *to be doing on the* (same date)*?"* You will often discover a great truth at this point: your client has absolutely no idea where he wants to go! Your job has suddenly become easier.

In all the above interventions, it is essential that you insist, coax, cajole or do whatever it takes to carry your client through to the completion. Pursue the idea you are working with until you are certain that everything has been 'taken on board'. Then change-work can commence.

Chapter 3

A Brief but Accurate Personality Test

This short test helps you to unobtrusively assess the basic personality group of your client, since the questions can be incorporated into conversation. If your client does not know she is being 'tested' the answers are likely to be more honest. This will allow you to choose the best possible induction for your client (see Chapter Eight) and will also help in the understanding of causes and origins of her symptom pattern(s). A comprehensive analysis of each group is given in the second part of this chapter.

Test and analysis

(1) If you had to choose, would you rather be rich or popular?

(2) And if you were rich, would you rather be quietly so, or evidently so?

(3) And where in your body do *you* actually 'live'?

The answers to these three questions can tell you an astonishing amount about your client. The one who chooses 'popular' will usually say she lives in her heart, thorax, or stomach. This is the Intuitive Adaptable (IA) personality, the responsive 'people person', governed by feelings, in touch with her emotions and easy to deal with in therapy, since she is usually quite suggestible and compliant. She tends to suffer emotional problems—low confidence, depressions, low self-esteem, etc. Her answer to question two may modify her personality categorisation a little as you will see later on, in the chart of possible combinations of answers. Almost any induction works well with this type.

The one who chooses 'rich, quietly' is likely to tell you she lives in her head. This is the Resolute Organisational (RO) personality, the intellectually-orientated, logical and analytical individual, governed by her thoughts rather than her feelings. She can be difficult for the inexperienced therapist because she tends to question everything. Interestingly, she is often fear-based and tends to suffer guilt complexes and phobic-type conditions, as well as anxiety over control issues. Hypochondria is not uncommon, nor is IBS (Irritable Bowel Syndrome). Care is needed with inductions, which must really grab her imagination and/or intellect. An effective method is to access one of her own vivid memories.

The one who would be 'rich, evidently' will tend to live in her **whole body,** or maybe not know what on earth you mean. This is the Charismatic Evidential (CE) type; she tends to be lively and noisy, though she is sometimes determinedly 'slob-like'. She can be an Actor (with a capital 'A') all the time, and *loves* attention. She is very likely to abreact in hypnosis and can be sobbing with evident anguish and then laughing 'like a drain' in the very next second. She is into self-gratification and pleasure, and tends to suffer from dramatic illnesses like spontaneous vomiting, violent rashes, severe diarrhoea, temper outbursts, frustration and the like. Alcohol dependence is common as are other forms of addiction. She usually goes into hypnosis 'at the drop of a hat' and responds best to novel induction methods like imagining vividly that her fingers are like hollow tubes, and that she can breathe in through her fingertips and out through her feet (or the other way around).

There are various combinations of answers:

Answer 1	Answer 2	Answer 3	Personality type
Popular	Quiet	Heart	IA
Popular	Quiet	Head	IA, but restrained, maybe inhibited (Some RO)
Popular	Quiet	Everywhere/ Don't know	IA, but unstable
Popular	Evident	Heart	IA, but outgoing (Some CE)
Popular	Evident	Head	Combination (see later)
Popular	Evident	Everywhere/ Don't know	CE acting IA
Rich	Quiet	Head	RO
Rich	Quiet	Heart	RO with a 'soft centre' (Some IA)

Rich	Quiet	Everywhere/ Don't know	Expressive RO (some CE)
Rich	Evident	Everywhere/ Don't know	CE
Rich	Evident	Head	CE, intellectually orientated (Some RO)
Rich	Evident	Heart	CE, emotionally/pleasure orientated (Some IA)

It is worth recognising that 'odd' or unusual answers to question (3) nearly always indicate the charismatic evidential personality, because the answers' qualities of novelty and differentness reflect those aspects of the CE type so well.

Personality types

Now we will have a detailed look at each of the three major personality types as revealed by this short test. No test, of course, is perfect, and the brevity of this one means that there may be those who do not seem to 'fit' what their answers suggest. Most of the time, though, it is astonishingly accurate. ***Remember that very few people will exhibit all the traits shown, due to the influence of the other groups.*** The combinations shown above will help you to understand this more easily.

Resolute Organisational

Personality Profile:

Forceful: Can always make their presence felt.

Resolute: High levels of tenacity and determination.

Organisational: Able to plan well and bring those plans to fruition.

Achilles heel: The need to always be in control.

25

Areas of conflict: Concerned with loss of respect/dignity/integrity or any sort of 'attack'—being frightened, picked on, humiliated, punished, bullied, accused, etc.

Abreaction type: Sometimes almost invisible—any tears are likely to be sparse, though this client may well feed as if she has been laid totally bare. The approach of abreaction will often be indicated by fear or anger.

Personality: RO personalities tend to have a reputation for firmness and a no-nonsense attitude to life. Psychologically stronger than either the IA or CE personality types, they find no difficulty in taking charge of things and easily attain the respect of others. They are cautious yet rapid thinkers who are unsurpassed at finding and exploiting the flaw in any argument. On the negative side, there can sometimes be a problem with cynicism and jealousy and there is not the immediately friendly response generally found in the IA. Indeed, there will sometimes be a significant pause before answering any question that is put to them and even then, the answer will often be carefully phrased in such a way as to leave as many options open as possible.

Positive attributes: Determined, tenacious, goal-orientated, methodical, perceptive, discreet, calm in emergencies, quick-thinking, practical and logical, good at recalling/using information to advantage.

Negative attributes: RO characters are inclined to force rather than subtlety and in negative mode are usually pedantic, domineering and impatient, and can appear rude and sarcastic. They have a driving need to be in control and can sometimes be quite ruthless in their determination to be so, being very good at manipulating people and events to advantage—which may, of course, be viewed as a positive trait under some circumstances. Cynicism or paranoia is usually evident. They hate not getting their own way, or having to admit that they are wrong.

Physical traits: This type is the least physically animated of the three groups. There are few changes of face expression during conversation, and few changes of body position. The angle of the head, in particular, may remain unchanged for longish periods making them reminiscent of an excellent card player, giving away absolutely nothing about inner thought processes. They appear to be—and indeed are—watchful and perceptive, with a steady gaze which may be away from their conversation partner if they are nervous. Any tension or anxiety will show in a taut body shape and a set facial expression leaning towards irritability or hostility.

Intuitive Adaptable

Personality Profile:

Sociable: Gets on well with almost anybody.

Intuitive: A high level of instinct and general awareness.

Adaptable: Able to make the best of any situation.

Achilles heel: The need to be liked.

Areas of conflict: Concerned with emotional states, predominantly guilt, shame, and injustice issues.

Abreaction type: Usually tearful and childlike. The approach of abreactive states will often be indicated by sudden quietness and an increase in hypnotic flush. A hand may be raised to the mouth, which may tremble or straighten. Tears and weeping can be copious.

Personality: The IA personality is a social chameleon, able to fit in with almost anybody or any situation. The most obvious traits are a pleasant and responsive attitude to others but sometimes with a tendency towards mood swings from happy to miserable—or the other way round—at the slightest provocation, the smallest event. There is also often an 'all or nothing' tendency, in which if they cannot have *absolutely* what they want, they will simply refuse to have any part of it at all and will 'cut off their nose to spite their face'. Excellent talkers and communicators, they are unrivalled when it comes to having an instinctive grasp of all that is going on around them. They are usually reliable and come over as 'nice' people, which they usually are.

Positive attributes: Instinctive understanding of others, communicative, caring, compassionate, persuasive, polite, usually cheerful, easy-going and tolerant, adaptable and versatile, can 'ride' disappointment.

Negative attributes: The complexity of this character can be truly exasperating; they can be just on the brink of success when they will suddenly give up on a plan or idea, claiming that they simply have not got what it takes, even if other people think they have. Feelings of inferiority and inadequacy can lead to problems with decision making and displays of under-confidence or unassertiveness, and they can take too much notice of the opinions of others, an excessive need to be liked sometimes leading to difficulty in saying "no" when necessary. There are often feelings of failure or of being in some way fraudulent. They are prone to shyness, depression and/or bouts of debilitating melancholia.

Physical traits: Responsive during conversation, with active but not excessive body/head movements, nodding when they should, smiling when they should, any disagreement being expressed politely and tactfully. Their facial expressions are reactive to the conversation and there is a tendency to smile often unless they are depressed. Any tension/anxiety present tends to speed up body movements and speech, and there will then be a leaning towards a worried/anxious expression.

IA personalities are the most complex of the three types; they will *always* have another influence present in the psyche; this is inevitable, since they are driven primarily by the dictates of the Superego (hence the wish to be popular, being the best person they can be) and the urges from the Id will not be completely denied. So there will be obvious traces of either one of the other two types, since *their* personalities are closer to the urges of the Id (control and survival in the case of the RO type, pleasure and gratification in the case of the CE type). This often shows, especially under pressure, as a very stubborn streak and a loathing of injustice in the IA/RO combination; and a bright and cheerful, sociable and outgoing disposition in the IA/CE combination.

Charismatic Evidential

Personality Profile:

Restless: Must always have something 'going on'.

Charismatic: Naturally outgoing.

Evidential: What-you-see-is-what-you-get.

Achilles heel: The need for constant stimulation.

Areas of conflict: Concerned with image issues and loss of freedom or things that they really did not want to do/face. These can seem to be quite minor events.

Abreaction type: Noisy and often may include screaming and shouting, as well as thrashing arms and legs—anything that *dramatically* illustrates how bad they are feeling. The approach of abreaction is usually rapid and almost indeterminable from the abreaction itself.

Personality: The CE personality in its purest form tends towards extremes in many things. CE personalities enjoy life to the full and can give much pleasure to a great many people along the way—except for the occasions when they get carried away with frivolity and excitement, loving to shock others with loud and embarrassing behaviour and being amazed when someone complains about their excesses. This exuberance tends to show itself quite often and can be quite exhausting/tiresome for their companions. Most of the time, though, this personality is tempered by more sensible traits from the other two groups, not unusually producing an individual who can quite often uplift others with their irrepressible sense of fun and enthusiasm.

Positive attributes: Enthusiastic, lively, inspirational, unsurpassable in publicity/promotion matters, confident and outgoing, uninhibited, good presentation skills, uncomplicated, fun-loving.

Negative attributes: The biggest problem for CE personalities is in maintaining application of effort, and as a result they can appear unreliable or fickle. They themselves are unconcerned about this, however, relying on sheer force of personality/charisma to see them through and usually getting away with it; they may even boast about it. There is a childish need for instant gratification—they cannot abide waiting about for things to happen—and a distinct tendency to flamboyantly exaggerate their successes. Their relationships are usually distinctly one-sided and they can be masters of tactlessness and bad taste, maybe even slob-like. Under pressure, they are prone to dramatic illnesses like paralysis, apparent blindness, 'black-outs', memory-loss, etc., which may or may not be genuine.

Physical traits: Animated behaviour is the most obvious trait here but, as with most things in this group, it tends to be exaggerated. There are excessive movements of the head and face, the body, and especially the hands, and they can liven up any gathering with sparkling wit—as long as not too much serious stuff is expected from them. Often quite generous and outgoing, and almost exclusively extroverts, they are always on the search for something new and exciting to do. They adore telling jokes and stories with lots of noise and action and almost always do it well. Under any sort of pressure, they tend to become louder and more expansive in their gestures and movements.

Combination personality

The somewhat rare combination personality—where there is an equal balance of all three groups—will be either:

(1) Extremely gifted and versatile, able to take on anything and succeed. May seem to lead an apparently charmed life.

(2) Prevaricating and anxious, always seeking to avoid responsibilities. Can seldom be assertive and may exhibit the 'doormat' syndrome.

You will notice that the two types are completely opposite—and there is seldom an in-between—one being a combination of the negative attitudes, the other enjoying an apparently effortless 'cruise' through the process of living. For those lucky people, everything seems to work out well, though, interestingly, they will not always recognise this for themselves and are not usually conceited or overbearing, usually taking some degree of pleasure in sharing their success. It is worth noting that the right sort of therapy can 'convert' the individual shown by (2), above, into something approaching that at (1), though their memory of what used to be will often prevent them from fulfilling their potential.

In positive mode, they are curious about many things and are often 'searchers for truth', actively investigating a great number of diverse concepts concerned with religion, para-psychology, culture, astrology and other forms of divination, as well as more practical matters such as the latest type of car engine. In short, they are interested in just about everything and have a better than average grasp of most that they observe.

The negative 'version' will, in fact, exhibit almost the same traits, except that they will show up as not being able to stick at anything, and will often end up as a defeated 'jack of all trades'. Their pre-conceptions tend to ensure that they misunderstand much of what they encounter.

Quick recognition guide

This brief guide will help you to recognise each type at a glance:

Resolute Organisational

Physiology: Fairly straight-faced, few body response patterns, steady gaze.

Positive: Practical, tenacious and self-sufficient. Quick thinkers.

Negative: Suspicious, dictatorial, manipulative. Cannot easily admit mistakes.

Dress: Plain, sometimes austere, sometimes tending towards dark colours.

Intuitive Adaptable

Physiology: Responsive body and head movements. Frequent smiles.

Positive: Caring, cheerful, pleasant, talkative and tolerant. 'People' people.

Negative: Depressive, indecisive, underconfident. Prone to mood swings.

Dress: Conservative, 'sensible', with a tendency to co-ordinate colours.

Charismatic Evidential

Physiology: Expansive in gestures. Can be animated/noisy. Laughs easily.

Positive: Fun-loving, enthusiastic, outgoing. Inspiring and optimistic.

Negative: Unreliable, childish, boastful. Prone to exaggerate mild success.

Dress: Individualistic, either 'designer' or deliberately downbeat. May be 'showy' with accessories.

This personality test and its associated assessments are accurate enough for you to be certain of a higher understanding of your client's *real* self than you might otherwise have gained.

Chapter 4

Preparing the Client (1)

Helping clients to understand exactly why a faulty belief system is at the bottom of their current difficulties is an important task for the therapist. As with all information, the cleaner and faster we can get it in, the easier and greater will be the understanding; the easier and greater the understanding, the more effective will be the therapy.

It is important to get therapy off to a 'flying start' because, otherwise, it can too easily actually become *a part of* your client's problems. To avoid that unhappy circumstance, you need to create change within the client even before he fully understands what the belief system actually is and what it does—almost before therapy starts, in fact. This is actually quite easy to do during the initial consultation, and what we are going to look at in this chapter is just one of the things you can do to start the process of change. There are other aspects of this elsewhere in the book and you can choose which to combine into your initial presentation of your therapy.

Many clients are convinced that they have at least *some* idea of why they are the way they are, why they cannot do the things they want to do, why they feel compelled to do things they do not want to do, etc. Others are not so sure, claiming that they have felt like they do for as long as they can remember, and will often look at you with an air of hopelessness, half expecting you to agree with their unspoken fear that it is 'just the way they are'. In either case, we need to grab their attention and hold it for as long as we can.

How about this:

> *"Well, I know **exactly** when your problem actually started… it was a long time ago. One hundred thousand years ago, to be exact."*

That usually grabs them; now all we have to do is *keep* them grabbed! While they are still considering the implications of what you have just said and attempting to work out what on earth you might mean, you continue with:

*"You see, when we are born, we're not born with a 'clean slate' as it were. A lot of people reckon we are and that it's only what happens to us after we're born that forms our personality. Well, you ask any mother who has more than one child, and she'll tell you that they were different from each other right at the very beginning, that they each had a personality in place already. You see, our particular species has been around for at least one hundred thousand years, maybe more, and it's over that period of time that the human way of being has developed. And considering that anything before about five thousand years ago is considered prehistoric—that is, before history started to be recorded—you can see that we have ninety-five thousand years of wandering savage in our make-up and only five thousand years of what we laughingly call civilisation. Not a surprise then, that we're born with some primitive behaviour patterns all ready and raring to go. You can think of those primitive behaviour patterns as Ancestral Memories, and since genetic inheritance seems to be random, it's quite easy for a child to be born to a parent who is quite different from him—or, to put it another way, we get the wrong parents. And then, of course, those parents are going to try to teach us a whole **load** of stuff that conflicts with what **we** are designed to be, even it suits **them**—which it probably doesn't half the time, anyway. So, those people who say that our personality is formed by what happens to us are right, in a way, but it's the conflicts that those events create, and the conflicts between what is right for us and what is right for those that teach us, that cause the problem. We're all different because we're **born** different and react to things differently. So we can be brought up in the same house with the same parents and so on, but be quite different from our brothers and sisters."*

This is a good time for a bit of interaction to ascertain that they have grasped the portent of your dissertation so far. Ask them if they have any experience of that effect of siblings being markedly different from each other, then draw their attention to the fact that identical twins tend to be strikingly similar in their way of being, even if they are brought up separately without knowing that the other exists. There have been several instances of this.

Continue with:

> *"It's all to do with what I call emotional stacks in your mind. You see, when you were born, you inherited a set of genes that equipped you to deal with certain amounts of emotion and behaviour. Not real stacks of course, just a convenient way of thinking of the way that emotion works. Let us take one of the most primitive of human emotions. Fear."*

Here, you could do a quick precis of the autonomic fight/flight instinctive response and the way it varies from one individual to another. Point out that what scares one person enough for him to run away, may simply spur someone else into some other sort of action. Of course, that situation exists in childhood, because each person is different. Then continue:

> *"Now, of course, when we are small, our emotional responses are far more profound than when we are adult, so something that causes a huge fright to a child will cause that fear stack to increase quite a bit. Now that stack—you can think of it as a pile coins if you like— doesn't just **measure** what we feel, it also **indicates** that we have discovered that there is some pretty scary stuff out there. And if that happens two or three times, well, that fear stack is going to get so big that we're going to search for fear in everything we encounter, because we'll believe there's more of that stuff about than anything else. So you can begin to understand why some people seem excessively nervous about things all the time, always looking for what can go wrong. Their childhood experiences have generated a stack of fear that is colouring their judgement of the world, and they have experienced more fear than they are designed to handle. And you can also begin to understand why something that affects one person so badly that he cannot function properly for a while afterwards, might leave another with hardly a raised eyebrow. But **that** individual would have a problem with something else, perhaps. Like the motorcycle racer who can take bends at 200mph with his knee half an inch off the ground, who nearly wets himself with terror when he has to speak at his best friend's wedding, for example."*

Let that sink in for a moment or two—ask your client if it all makes sense so far. It is important not to progress too fast, because we need our client to fully understand where we are going. In any case, you would have spent only a few minutes on this concept at this point. When you are ready, continue:

> *"Now, supposing, just supposing, we could take of a pile of coins from that fear stack and chuck 'em away! Well, actually, they don't get thrown away, because they represent energy and you can't destroy energy. What actually happens to those coins is they get put back where they came from in the first place… the confidence stack. We don't lack confidence when we are born. How can we? We lose it as a result of things happening to us."*

Your client will usually have become very interested by now, because the one thing that every one of your clients will have in common is a lack of confidence in some way. It may be general or it might be contained in one phobic reaction like flying, for instance; but wherever it is, they will have that lack of confidence. It is why they are sitting in front of you. Continue:

> *"Now, as it happens, we **can** actually do something very like that. We can actually find a way of letting go of some of the fear that's been stored up in that stack. And we can get that energy back into the confidence stack. Of course, it might be other emotions as well, but almost everybody has fear in some way, even if it's just a bit of low self-confidence. Now, shall I tell you how we can do that?"*

Wait for the client's response—which is always a 'yes' of some sort—and any questions, before you tell him about your particular mode of working. It creates a high belief set for analysis, regression, guided imagery, visualisation, suggestion… just about any type of therapeutic endeavour.

If you are using anything other than analysis, regression or some other form of 'uncovering' therapy, then that is pretty much as far as you need to go, as far as setting up your client is concerned. It is a fairly safe bet that, by now, he has a subconscious awareness that he is not going mad; that his problem is probably not his fault; that a solution is possible; and that you know how to help him find it.

This manner of setting up the client works well for any type of therapeutic endeavour but it is the analytical/regression therapies that will probably benefit the most. This is because you now have a perfect 'tool' to persuade your client to tell you absolutely *everything* without hesitation, even those 'little' memories that he might otherwise have felt were too insignificant or irrelevant to bother you with. Every working therapist is very much aware that those particular memories so often lead directly to the source of the presenting problem. In addition to this, there will be less hesitation about recounting the more embarrassing or shameful recalls, or those that have a good dollop of personal guilt attached.

Now, for those of you who earnestly believe that there is never any need or justification to have a client tell us these personal things, we are not saying here that it *is* essential, or that the client will not get better without doing this. What we are saying is if that is the way you work (and if you do then you will be just as certain of your belief as are those of the 'no need to tell' school) it will now be easier. You can explain that whenever an event takes place, the input from our senses affects each and every one of our stacks of emotional response, not just the major ones. Every one of them has been adjusted literally *millions* of times during our life and often, when we were young, those adjustments could be quite profound. This is why children will sometimes take an idea 'on board' (usually a negative one) quite abruptly, leaving parents and others wondering what on earth has happened. Now, of course, everything your client remembers and tells you about *instantaneously* adjusts each stack that was affected by that happening. Fear, guilt, joy, confidence, self-worth, love, assertiveness, aggression, anger, shame… all of them will be adjusted according to the *adult* relevance of each recall. The statement to use, fairly emphatically and dramatically is:

> *"So, you see, **every single thing** you tell me is going to lead you one step closer to your being the best person you can possibly be. **Every single thing** you tell me, little by little, is going to remove coins from the negative stacks and replace them in the confidence stack where they belong. So you steadily become more and more confident as you move closer and closer to the time when you can be the person you deserve to be. And all you have to do is make quite certain that you tell me every single thing that you remember. Will you do that?"*

Here, you *must* get a 'yes' from your client. If you do not, then there is a need to discover why and deal with that particular problem, which may be a need to defend somebody, his own embarrassment or guilt or whatever. Getting a 'yes' from your client also conditions him into the recognition that he is going to have to do at least some of the work himself. Note that it is important to get that 'yes' response to the question shown: "Will you do that?" rather than the apparently similar 'polite' alternative: "Do you think you can do that?"

An individual may very well decide he *can* do that—but it does not mean that he is agreeing that he *will*!

Chapter 5

Preparing the Client (2)

With any form of therapy, what you do with your client in the initial consultation and the first working session will govern the way that therapy proceeds. Obviously, it is important that your client must gain the impression that you are a total professional, properly trained, competent, and experienced at dealing with her particular problem.

But it goes deeper than that. It is necessary for you to 'tune' the processes of the subconscious so that they are orientated towards the likely source of problems, otherwise you could be in for a long haul. The same applies even if you are not using a regression style of therapy; if you can get the client's subconscious focused around the area of her psyche where the problem is, then any suggestion or guided imagery work you carry out will have a far greater chance of being successful.

During the initial consultation, these three areas of questioning will do a lot to start the process:

(1) Details of the presenting symptom(s).

(2) What the client wants therapy to achieve.

(3) What she feels is stopping her from achieving it on her own.

As far as question (1) is concerned, what the symptom is, how long it has existed, and what the client believes to be the cause of it are all obviously essential information.

Question (2) is important because it tells us whether the client has realistic expectations of what we can do, or if, instead, she is hoping for some sort of 'magic' to be performed. We should never be satisfied with a straightforward "I want to get rid of my symptom" type of answer; the client should be encouraged to tell us how she wants to be, how she wants to feel, what she wants to be able to do that she cannot do now. For many, this may be the first time they have directly addressed this particular aspect of their difficulties and it therefore focuses their mind on what they want to achieve. It is also an encouragement for them to look forward beyond their difficulties, to perceive that there may be an end in sight.

Question (3) tells us something of the resources that we need to help our client find. If what she tells us seems congruent with the answers to questions (1) and (2), all is well and we can soon begin to start work. It may be, though, that what she tells us here seems to be transparently inappropriate. In this case, we can attempt to elicit the *real* reason she believes she needs help, and when we are convinced she is telling us the truth as she perceives it, we should respect that it is the operative part of what she perceives to be her difficulty in life. If there is still a lack of congruence, *we can assume that this one is the only question she has answered fully so far* and ask more questions about her symptom(s) or her aspirations until we find out what is missing.

If we do not ascertain exactly where she is and where she wants to go, then neither we nor she will know when she has got there! For many people, simply defining full answers to those three questions can give them a much-needed sense of direction and put them on the road to recovery even before we have done any real work.

Obviously there would be more to the initial consultation, depending on the type of therapy you intend to use for any particular client. But once you get on to the first actual working session, it is a valid idea if you are working with any form of anxiety state or phobic pattern to make the entire session over to the rest of the 'setting up' process shown here, whatever your chosen method. The script works particularly well; it is advisable to keep precisely to the wording of the sections printed in bold, unless you are truly very experienced and know what you are doing. It is designed to gently guide the subconscious to a particular point in time, even though neither you nor the client has any idea at the outset about where that point in time is. You will see that it is orientated towards the 'talking' therapies of analysis and regression, but it is easily adapted for any type of therapeutic method.

Commence with any pre-talk or preparation before going on into whatever sort of induction will best suit your client's personality (see Chapter Three) and once you have your client into a nicely hypnotised state continue with:

"Now you're so beautifully relaxed... just allowing your thoughts to drift... all the way back... all the way back to those childhood years... those years between when you were born and finally made it to maturity... and for some people, maturity is as early as fifteen or so, while for others it may be as late as seventeen or even eighteen... just letting your mind drift all the way back to those years, when there was you, and there were the others... things they didn't understand... things you didn't understand... that time of private thoughts and fears and those secrets... when everything was so very new... when everything was so very new and all for the first time... when you were still finding out and discovering all the things you could do... and the things you couldn't do... and the things you weren't supposed to do, but did anyway... just letting your mind drift all the way back to those years... not searching for anything in particular, not questioning what you find there... but just allowing your subconscious mind to go where it needs to go...

"And I don't know whether you'll see pictures in your mind's eye... pictures that can sometimes be so vivid, so real, that it's just as if you're looking out through your forehead, so that what you saw then you can see again now, and what you felt then, you can feel again now... or maybe you'll just find yourself thinking thoughts, just remembering... or perhaps just feelings will come into your mind and body... feelings or pictures, or just thoughts and memories... or maybe even nothing at all, for some of the time... and whatever happens is right for you, because your subconscious, that powerful and all-knowing subconscious of yours, knows exactly what's right for you... so whatever happens, it's exactly what should happen... for you... exactly the right thing, without you searching for anything in particular, just allowing your mind to drift to wherever it wants to go... and because you have to do absolutely nothing at all, you simply cannot get it wrong... so you can be easy in your mind that whatever you find yourself thinking and feeling, it's the right thing to think and feel...

"And now I wonder if you can just let your mind drift around those early years, just remembering how things could seem so upsetting sometimes, back then... so upsetting that you can perhaps almost feel that same feeling again now... in your mind... or maybe even in your body... maybe sadness... or anger... or any of those other emotions that you could sometimes feel so sharply when you were just a child... in those years before maturity... jealousy, perhaps, or frustration... or feelings of being left out of things... and now I'd like you to reach down into wherever your memories are stored and gather up one of those times from the past... and tell me what it is you find yourself thinking of, the very first thing you find that comes up into your mind..."

Wait, urge, guide if necessary.

"Good, that's very good... now we're going to use a process called... free association... to let your subconscious mind link that memory up to any other memory that it knows is somehow connected... and all you have to do is just to allow that first memory to simply drift away... even push it away... and allow another thought to take its place or maybe reach down again into wherever your memories are stored and grab the first thing you find...without consciously trying to make any connection at all... and again, I want you to tell me what you find yourself thinking of..."

Wait, urge, guide if necessary.

"That's good... and all you have to do every time you come to see me is just that... just exactly what you did there, just then... and whatever you find yourself thinking is absolutely the right thing for you to think... whatever it is, however silly it seems to you, or however embarrassing it seems... **and sometimes people suddenly find themselves thinking of something absolutely awful that happened to them... something absolutely awful... that upset them so much at the time, they thought their whole world would never be right again... back there, back then, in those childhood years (pause)... and, of course, it's all right to feel again the emotions that went with those things... all right to feel any emotion that's still there, in the subconscious, stuck there since those childhood days...**

"And there were so many things that could happen to a child... unpleasant things sometimes, things that the grown-ups maybe knew absolutely nothing about... things that other children did (pause) ... things that other grown-ups did (pause) ... some things that were games which went wrong (pause) ... or just confusing things that you didn't quite understand (pause) ... things that left you feeling uncomfortable or bewildered, or sometimes hopelessly lost or completely alone ... and maybe even sometimes leaving you in an unfamiliar place, with unfamiliar people all around you (pause) ... and there's sometimes fear, too, back there in those child-hood years ... fear when it seemed there was something that was just too big to deal with all on your own (pause) ...

"And just about now you might suddenly find yourself thinking about something that you really wish you had not thought about at all ... that guilty secret ... a guilty secret you've kept quiet about for years and years that suddenly seems to fill your mind so much that ... there's nothing else there for a moment or two ... fills your mind so much that it seems to you that I must surely realise exactly what you're thinking ... a guilty secret that you'd give just about anything to keep quiet so that nobody found out ..."

All of the foregoing, especially the bold section, which should not be vocally emphasised during the session, has been leading up to and preparing the client for what we are about to do now:

"But all those things back there, in those childhood years, are just memories now ... and it's safe to remember those things ... because they are from a long time ago, when you were just a child ... and I wonder if you can see yourself looking just as you did when you were a small child ... just make a vivid picture in your mind of you as a small child ... and now I want you to do a really clever, very special trick ... I want you, as an adult, to reach back through time ..."

Whichever of the following you continue with depends on how well you feel your client can react. Although (2) is best, some people, in particular RO males (see Chapter Three), tend to 'freeze' on it. In those cases, start with (1) and observe the reaction—if it is evident, then go on to (2).

(1) *"... and just be there with that small child for a few moments... just being there and offering comfort in any way you can... offering comfort so that that small child just knows that it's okay ... that it's safe to remember now... that it's all right to tell now...*

(2) *"... and give that small child a hug ... just reach back through time as an adult and give that child a hug ... and just say: 'It's all right ...' to that small child (pause) ... just say: 'Everything's all right ... it's safe to remember, now ... all right to tell, now ...' (pause)"*

Be ready with the tissues at this point and allow enough time for your client to 'focus'. By far the vast majority will hit an emotional response which may well be profound. The next section could be changed to incorporate whatever suggestion or imagery work you wish/need to use.

"And now you can let your mind drift away from the past ... coming back to the here and now, coming back up to date, back to this room, to the here and now, with the speed of an express train so that all those memories and feelings are not only years behind, but thousands upon thousands of miles behind, too ... so that you can leave behind any unpleasant feelings we disturbed today ... just leaving them here with me, when you go ... and next time you come to see me, it's going to be twice as easy to be twice as relaxed ... easy to remember things ... easy to tell me the things you remember ... but in the meantime, you'll find yourself with all sorts of flashbacks to those childhood years ... all sorts of little memories occurring to you, just when you least expect it ... and sometimes in dreams, too ... and you'll find that you remember your dreams and you can write those dreams down and bring them to me the next time you come to see me ...

"Next time you come to see me, it's going to be twice as easy to be twice as relaxed, easy to remember things, easy to tell me things... but in the meantime, you're going to find yourself with a good feeling of being at ease within yourself... when you close my door behind you as you leave, you're going to find yourself with a good feeling, a feeling that it's all going to be all right... in fact, you're going to find that things that used to upset you are going to now just calm and relax you, and the more they could previously upset you, the more they're going to now just simply calm and simply relax

you… so that all the things you used to have trouble in dealing with are going to seem so easy to you from now on, you'll find yourself wondering if they were ever truly a problem in the first place … so easy to you from now on, you'll find yourself being an inspiration to other people … and that feels good …

"And next time you come to see me, it's going to be easier to relax, easy to remember things, easy to tell me things … just knowing within yourself that you're going to tell me everything you remember, and everything you tell me will lead you one step closer to the time when you can be … exactly as you wish to be … one step closer to you being … the best person you can be.

"And now it's time for me to bring the session to an end …"

It is not at all unusual for your client to arrive for her second working session reporting that she feels far more comfortable with herself than she can remember feeling for a long time. Some clients will have had vivid dreams, even nightmares, via which the subconscious has sought—maybe even successfully—to discharge the underlying anxiety. Just occasionally, a client might report feeling far worse than she did to begin with; this is still good news from the therapy point of view, since it is evidence that the process of change has started. The fact that this initial change is not particularly beneficial should not concern us one iota; it is the end result we seek, and your client's subconscious is now ready and raring to go!

Chapter 6

Preparing the Client (3)—the Private Place

This script can be incorporated into your initial induction. Commence your induction in the most appropriate way and take your client to 10 steps leading down to a beautiful garden. Now continue as follows:

"And just imagine now taking your very first step on the cool, green, velvety grass. The sun is high in the sky and it's the clearest blue sky you have ever seen. The warmth of the sun feels good on your skin and a gentle breeze carries the fragrance of many flowers in the air. Everything here is growing just as nature intended. No one else for miles and miles and miles, just you and the sound of my voice. As you lazily stroll through the garden, all around you are trees, bushes, shrubs and flowers... flowers of the most vibrant colours you have ever seen... some of them in beautifully designed flowerbeds and some growing wherever the seed has landed, perhaps carried on the breeze. Notice there your favourite flower, enjoy and marvel at its luxurious petals and the strong stem supporting the delicate bloom, all of the plant being nourished from deep within the rich earth as the roots reach down and create balance.

"In the distance you can see a stream... and as you walk towards it you begin to hear the sounds of the water travelling on its way perhaps to a brook or a river or to some far distant ocean. Stand for a moment and just watch the crystal clear water, fresh and gleaming in the sunshine... As you look at the surface it is an illusion, for at just the right place and at just the right time you'll notice the pebbles beneath the water shining and sparkling like gems, emeralds, sapphires, diamonds and rubies.

"Look around you and breathe in the fresh air easily and naturally. You feel good in this place, still and quiet inside... On the far side of the stream you can see rolling green hills and mountains, some so high they have snow on top. The sunshine shimmers on the snow, looking like hundreds of twinkling, dancing lights, and you can wonder if perhaps the stream began its journey high up in those

mountains, always following its path, nothing stopping its natural flow.

"Further downstream you notice a small, stone bridge crossing over the water and as you make your way along the side of the stream towards the bridge, you notice as you stroll that you feel more and more peaceful inside, and discover a carefree feeling of well-being. Some trees are growing near the bridge and their branches reach over towards the water, the rays of sunlight streaming through the branches and dancing on the water... As you get closer and closer to the bridge you begin to see the moss and grass growing through the cracks making its way lazily towards the sun. Step safely on to the bridge and make your way to the other side of the stream, hearing the sound of the water gently splashing as it continues on its journey. On this side of the bridge there are 3 steps leading down to a door and you can see a soft light shining beneath the door... the light has a very warm and welcoming sense about it.

"Notice the colour of the door and see your name written on the door in gold... this is your private place where no one else may enter, just you and the sound of my voice. Imagine going down the steps now— three, two, one, zero. That's right... you notice the door opens in a way that is characteristic of you."

Pause for approximately 5 seconds.

"Gently open the door. Feel the soothing sensation of the light and enter your private place, be sure to close the door behind you so no one else may enter.

"On your left is a full-length mirror with a very distinctive frame and something else you notice is that it has a pink glow—a sort of fluorescent pink glow—very unusual and different...One wall is full of bookshelves with so many different books—big books, little books, hardbacks, paperbacks, different colours, some leather-bound. But there's one book in particular which takes your attention...one book in particular takes your attention, because you notice it has your name written on it... Notice its colour, see how your name is written. Just notice it there on the shelf.

"On another wall there's a screen, like a cinema screen, it's the size of the entire wall and it glows silvery in the light—there's nothing to see on the screen at this time. You glance around and notice that close by the screen is the most unusual video-player you have ever seen but you can't quite make out what it is that's different, just yet. Notice everything. See there on the shelf a picture of yourself as you are right now, as you are at this moment in time.

"Look at the floor, perhaps it is carpeted, or tiled, maybe it's earth or wood. Notice the colour, feel the sensation beneath your feet and notice the large white circle there in the design on the floor.

"Look at the ceiling and just make a note of what you see ... On the wall nearest the bookshelves there is what looks like a large letterbox about the size of a rubbish-chute hatch. You know the sort of heavy, metal letterbox you see on the outside of a bank, which has a strong handle to pull down and open. Just see it there in your room ... and know that it's there ... because, feeling quite drowsy now, you just want to relax. Move into your room a little further and notice the very relaxing and comfortable chair. Move the pillows and cushions, fluff them up just how you would like them to be and relax even more as you sit in the warmth and safety of your private place.

"On the left arm of the chair is the remote control for the video. On one side it looks like any other remote control but if you pick it up and turn it over, that's right, see there it has a QWERTY keyboard ... the same sort of keyboard you find on typewriters and computers ... On your right-hand side is a low table. It looks like a coffee table, and on top of the table are some boxes ... all different—different sizes, different colours, some hand-painted, some decorated with bright, sparkly jewels, some varnished and some plain. Just notice them there on the table. Also on the table is a bunch of keys, notice them just lying there by the boxes.

"Next to the boxes is the telephone. It looks quite ordinary really just like any other telephone but look again because you'll notice there are no numbers, that's right, there are no numbers on this telephone. Let your gaze drift back again to the boxes on the table, the remote control with the QWERTY keys, the silver screen shimmering on the wall. Notice again the video-player, the rubbish-chute in the wall ... the shelves, the books...notice again the book with your name on it

... and that beautiful pink, glowing mirror with the distinctive frame... the white circle on the floor. Take a moment and notice— familiarise yourself with this room."

Pause for approximately 10 seconds.

"Now very slowly and lazily begin to stand up and walk across the room towards the door. Stand by the door and look back into your private place. We shall return here again and you will always notice something different. Every time you return here you will always notice something to your advantage. You may not always recognise it at first but you will know it when you need to.

"Step outside now and close the door. It feels good to be out in the sunshine. Up the 3 steps towards the bridge. It is time to leave this place now. Going over the bridge, pause for a moment in the middle of the bridge and watch the flow of the water, hear the sound of the leaves in the trees as the gentle breeze drifts through the branches, notice again the wonderful fragrances of the plants and flowers. Feel good just... being."

This is a good time for suggestions for a positive outcome to therapy, etc.

"Continuing over the bridge now and—stepping on to the path— you notice the different textures beneath your feet as you stroll along by the water's edge.

"Leaving the path now, step on to the soft velvety grass, move past the flowerbeds, up through the garden towards the steps."

Now close the session in the most appropriate way.

There are many benefits to incorporating the 'private place' into your first session of hypnosis. It prepares your client for some of the other techniques in this book, the bunch of keys and the telephone to mention but two. But the real beauty of it is that if you decide that you need some sort of device/tool for your client to use in his imagination, he will always find it in this private place. When you have taken him there, you can simply follow with: *"and as you look around you, you realise that, although you've never noticed it before, there's a... "*

Chapter 7

The Excessively Logical, Analytical or Resistant Client

Our purpose here is not to conduct an in-depth look at the whole area of resistance issues—it would take a whole book, and much has already been written on the subject. Most readers will already be familiar with 'tricks' like pacing and leading, establishing rapport, exploring modalities, and the like.

The purpose of this chapter is to give you a couple of easy methods to get certain of your clients on the right track and to give you at least a fair chance of establishing a good work situation.

One of the major problems when dealing with the excessively logical/analytical type of personality is getting her to understand that she actually *can* suspend logical thought and allow her imagination to be used in a constructive manner. This serves three important purposes:

(1) It allows her to accept that her mind can respond to suggestion.

(2) It makes it easier to get her into a decent working state of hypnosis.

(3) It automatically lowers resistance levels.

You will quickly see that what is presented here is nothing more than two suggestibility tests, but when they are presented in the way they are here, it is very rare indeed for somebody to 'fail' **both** of them. If a client does, it is evidence either that we have work to do before getting her anywhere near the hypnosis chair/couch, or that we might want to think again before taking her into therapy. At best, she is likely to be less than obliging; at worst, downright awkward.

The logical/analytical client is usually seeking to be in control; she views us, albeit subconsciously—perhaps—as being on 'the other side of the fence' from her, and therefore to be resisted in the way she would resist an opponent in an argument. It is even possible that she will be seeking to maintain her symptom because of a hidden agenda, because she finds change threatening, or because she does not want the therapist to be able to do something that she cannot.

*So we have to do something to help her to recognise the truth that we are working **with her**, and not for ourselves. And that is a very important distinction, of course.*

Much of this can be achieved by standard methods of rapport building but being able to show her how she can use the powers of her own mind will often work wonders for her.

Test one

Begin by saying: "All right. Before we do anything else, I'd like to establish just how powerful your mind actually is." Then ask her to pinch thumb and forefinger together and show her exactly what you mean. Then, holding your own thumb and forefinger together, run the tip of your other forefinger around the outside of the join between them as you say: "Now, I'd like you to imagine that somebody has put Superglue or something like it between them… that you can actually **feel** that they are stuck together. Just pretend that they are stuck tight together, and while you're pretending that they're stuck absolutely tight together, see if you can open them."

Now, here is the important thing: MOST PEOPLE **WILL** OPEN THEIR FINGERS, because most people's *conscious critical faculty* will tell them that their fingers are most certainly *not* stuck together. That is exactly what this test is designed for—failure. You have actually led them to fail (though it is doubtful that they'll notice it) by the provocative suggestion/implication that their mind must be strong to be able to 'overcome' your suggestion—or the suggestion that they *think* you made that their fingers should remain stuck tightly together.

Now you smile and say: "Ah, good!" and pause for just a moment or two before you continue: "Now, there, you thought about the fingers opening instead of being stuck together, and of course, they opened. Now, in the same way, if you think of something happening and if your mind and your imagination is strong enough for you to imagine it really well and believe it, then your mind will try to make it happen." Wait for this to sink in, then continue: "Now I wonder if you can use your mind *that* powerfully with imagining something different." Of course, they are now in a perfect double bind which they may or may not realise: on the next test, they can prove that their mind *is* strong by using their imagination to succeed with the test, or they can prove that it is not by failing! What they will definitely have begun to realise by now is that there is nothing magical about to go on, just that they are going to use their own mind power for themselves and that you are not going to do all the work. *Plus* they have observed that you have not been at all 'phased' by something happening which they perceived as being opposite to that which you expected. They have already learnt that they cannot read the therapist's mind and that if they offer resistance, they may actually be doing exactly what you wanted.

Of course, if they do not open their fingers, simply praise them and tell them (because it's true) that they are able to use their imagination more powerfully than most people can. In this case, there is no need for you to perform the following test unless you especially want to, because your client is already conditioned to allow the conscious critical faculty to be bypassed. You can begin any hypnotic induction or suggestion sequence and know that the client is going to be compliant.

Otherwise, you move on.

Test two

This time, ask the client to extend the forefinger of her major hand and make it stiff—and show her what you mean. It is better if you have your finger pointing up towards the ceiling. Once she has done this, ask her if she has ever seen those army/scout knives with a steel spike that is used for getting stones out of horses hooves, or something similar. If she has, good, if not, ask her to just imagine a solid, thick, pointed steel spike, as thick as her finger and shiny and rigid. While you are doing this, just pinch each knuckle of your extended finger between the thumb and forefinger of your other hand, while saying: "Now, I'd like you to imagine that that finger is as stiff and rigid as that steel spike, that the knuckles simply **cannot** bend… in fact, I'd like you to imagine that that finger is so stiff and sharp, that you could **plunge** it through a panel door." As you say '**plunge**', illustrate the action of plunging your own forefinger through an imaginary panel. Then continue: "Now, while you're imagining that, see what happens if you try to bend that finger—but make sure you're imagining it to be as rigid as that steel spike." It is important that you use that phrase, 'see what happens if you try to bend that finger' as it is here, because the semantics are important.

The vast majority of your clients will bend the finger from the knuckle on the hand only, so that the finger remains stiff. Some will struggle and not even move the finger at all. Either way, you instantly congratulate them and tell them to relax the finger now, because they have proved what you both knew—that they have an **excellent** mind and imagination. Go gently as you point out that they could easily have bent the finger if they had really wanted to, so they have also discovered just how easy it is to use the power of their mind to overcome their logical self—the part of self that might have actually tried to defeat them in their efforts to become well.

Now, of course, you are going to find any suggestion of eye closure/lock is far more likely to be complied with, for they will instantly recognise that you are requiring them to *imagine how it would be* if their eyes were locked tightly shut. They will know how to do it and they will know that succeeding in this is demon-strating, once again, the strength of their mind. They have nothing to prove now and they are instantaneously approaching a working state of hypnosis.

Where an individual 'fails' that second test, you can be reasonably certain that there is a **lot** of resistance present, because it is actually easier to keep the finger stiff than it is to bend it, and she should by now *want* it to work. You will need to find a way to resolve that resistant state before continuing with therapy, otherwise you could find yourself with a client who can scarcely wait to tell you, each time she comes to see you, that she is not improving.

When that second test *is* failed, you could do a lot worse than responding with: "That's interesting! Why did you do that?" Your client is likely to reply along the lines of "Well, I tried and it bent," or something similar. You would then need to pursue that same line about getting her mind to work *for* her, instead of against her. Tactfully point out that what is happening is that the part of her mind which has not made much of a job of getting her better (otherwise why is she with you?) is interfering with the part of the mind which *will* help her—the creative and imaginative part. "We have to discover if you are able to use that part of your mind effectively enough for therapy to work properly," is a good phrase.

Most of the time, your client will at least pay lip-service to an understanding, in which case she is moving towards compliance. But it may be that, in spite of your best efforts, she stubbornly refuses to accept that her logic is getting in the way, and just as stubbornly refuses to accept that by-passing logical resistance will get her to where she wants to be. In this case, you may be best not taking this particular client into therapy.

This 'why did you do that?' response is actually very useful on other occasions; for example, when a client opens her eyes in the middle of an induction, or suddenly decides to sit up, or demonstrates some other version of 'Look, look! I'm not hypnotised!'

Because there is not really a sensible answer to: 'Why did you do that?' the response is quite often an embarrassed grin and apology, and a return to the previous state. Then you continue as if nothing has happened and make no mention of it unless the client does. Even then, treat it as unimportant. Now we'll have a look at some of the other possible responses:

Client: *Because I'm not hypnotised.*

Response: *Tell me how hypnosis feels.*

Of course, if she tells you the truth—that it feels no different to a normal state of 'eyes closed, relaxing in a chair' you ask her how she felt different and take it from there. If she tells you, as is usually the case, that she should be semi-conscious, 'out of it', going to sleep or whatever, ask her who taught her that this should be the case and again take it from there. If she insists that she is right and you are wrong, then, as with an earlier example, you might as well discharge her from therapy there and then, because you are into a conflict situation which is unlikely to be satisfactorily resolved.

> **Client:** *Because I couldn't see the (stairs/beach/room/hill/lake or whatever it was you were suggesting)*

> **Therapist:** *Okay, that's all right. You can just think of it, instead, and imagine how it would be if you could see it."*

> **Client:** *Because I didn't like the feeling I got.*

> **Therapist:** *Splendid! Let's investigate that—it's bound to be part of your problem.* (This, of course, is absolutely true. Pursue it, and seek to find out when she first felt that way.)

> **Client:** *Because I wanted to.*

> **Therapist:** *And you wanted to do that because...?* (Pursue this avenue until it is exhausted. 'Don't know' is not a valid answer.)

> **Client:** *Well, I just could.*

> **Therapist:** *Okay. But I wonder... now that I know that you **can** do that, can your mind be strong enough to **resist** doing that?*

Notice that in all cases, you are actually working *with* the resistance and not obviously seeking to overcome it in some way. The last response is a fairly complete double bind, which is an effective way of working: your client is placed in the situation where she can choose to go along with what you are asking her to do, or admit that her mind is not as strong as she thought.

This list is not exhaustive, but it will give you a good idea of how you might easily overcome what might otherwise be a time-wasting and distinctly non-therapeutic situation.

Continued resistance

It is rare, if you handle the initial consultation properly and incorporate the tests shown earlier where necessary, that you will find yourself with a client who is exhibiting an absolutely determined resistance. Rare, but it *will* happen sometimes. Usually there is a hidden agenda at work, or maybe a secondary gain. This is a different situation from that which exists with the types who are just anxious to prove that *you* cannot 'get' *them*.

The hidden agenda is simply a reason that the client has to maintain the state she is in. A depressed individual, for example, may not wish to become cheerful, because she would receive less support from friends and family. This process is likely to be almost or completely unconscious, and the fact that she would not *need* that support from others if she were well is being completely overlooked. In this case, the client is projecting forwards the thought of how it would be **now**, while she is still suffering depression, if people were leaving her to fend for herself some of the time. A simple illustration of the power of this sort of subconscious process is the well-known circumstance that a supermarket shopper will buy more food for the store cupboard if she is hungry while shopping. She is basing future requirements on how she feels *now*.

The secondary gain is slightly different from the hidden agenda, in that the client here has a distinct *benefit* to be derived from not becoming well. Litigation in progress after an accident would be a very powerful secondary gain for not becoming well, especially if there is a large amount of money involved. The client is more likely to be aware of this mental process than she would be with the hidden agenda, but no more likely to admit it.

When the hidden agenda exists, the client wishes to remain ill; when a secondary gain is existent, the client does not want to become well. The situations are subtly different but you will need to help the client resolve either before therapy can be of any real help. To this end, a fair bit of 'detective' work might be necessary.

In these situations, indeed in all resistance situations, there are certain client behaviours to watch out for. You can never *defeat* resistance and any attempt to do so will simply fuel it and make it stronger, so you have to go with it. One of the commonest problems is illustrated in a 'will to power' situation where the client seeks to in some way get control of the therapist. Here are some examples:

Client: *I'm making this session my last one.* (This is seeking to empower her by making you have to 'chase' her. Go with it.)

Therapist: *Good, I'm really glad you're feeling well enough to stop.* (The client may well come back with "I'm not! I'm just not getting better" or something similar. The only way to deal with that is to say something like: "Oh, I see. Well, of course, it's all right for you to get in touch with me if you want to pick it up again.")

Client: *I need to come in on* (a time when you wouldn't normally be there) *this week or I shall have to miss my session.* (Again, seeking to empower her by getting control of your work hours. Go with it.)

Therapist: *Well, it's better if you don't miss, but I can't do that time so I'll book you for the same time next week?* (It is amazing how frequently clients decide they can probably make it, after all.)

Client: *Your therapy isn't working. I'm not getting better.*

Therapist: (with a smile) *No, it's **your** therapy, not mine. What would you like to do?*

Client: (with apparent triumph) *I'm sorry, I definitely didn't go under! No way!*

Therapist: *Okay … but could you tell me what it is that pleases you about not being able to enter hypnosis? It will help your therapy enormously if you can understand what's happening there.*

Client: *Your therapy hasn't worked and I want my money back!*

Therapist: *I've applied the correct therapy for you, so I can't make a refund. But I will give you the address of my trade association if you* *want to take it up with them.* (The client may threaten to sue, or expose you as a fraud in the media or some other such threat, but giving in to any of this is unprofessional and *an admission that you are at fault, which could have repercussions later on.* Your response should remain as above.)

Client: *I don't want you to do what you've suggested. I want you to* (reference to something that a friend or relative 'had done' or something she's seen on television or a stage show or read somewhere.)

Therapist: *Well, there are all sorts of methods of therapy, and any therapist worth his salt will only work in the way that he is happy with. So would you like me to work as I've suggested?*

You will observe that the common factor in all the above is that the onus remains with the client. Even where a refund is being demanded, the therapist's response is to refuse to enjoin in 'battle'.

There are many other forms that resistance might take; but this chapter should have given you a few ideas to help deal with them.

Chapter 8

Choosing the Right Induction for Your Client

Choosing the right induction for your client's personality type is of considerable importance. Whilst it is certainly true that a progressive relaxation will induce *most* people into a working state of hypnosis, it will not necessarily produce the *best* state of hypnosis that they can achieve. This chapter outlines the type of work that the three main personality groups will best and most quickly respond to; there is no need to rely on the boredom factor of monotony.

Each induction shown here assumes some sort of preparation phase, a short *'settle down and make yourself comfortable'* routine.

The resolute organisational type

This personality type tends to march to his own tune somewhat and will automatically subconsciously resist anything which is perceived to leave another individual in control. The best way to produce a good state of hypnosis here is to actually *use* his own control-orientated, intellectually-based thinking processes. Forget relaxation—this may be perceived as faintly ridiculous or even 'soft' and, in any case, the fact that you are telling him that **you want** him to relax can place him immediately on 'alert status'.

If you want a good result here, it is necessary to engage your client's thought processes as rapidly as possible, ideally in a way which is impossible to resist. Logical work works well and the following is one of the best examples of this. It incorporates a start routine that is reminiscent of the work of Dave Elman.

The mental map

> *"All right, I'd like you now to just close your eyes... just close your eyes and allow your eyelids to be just as relaxed and heavy as you would like them to be... just as heavy and relaxed as you would choose them to be... if you can use the power of your own mind to*

relax them to the point where you can easily pretend that they simply will not work, or that they are just a single sheet of skin, that's fine... but if you can't get them quite as relaxed as that, that's fine, too... just allow them to be as relaxed, just as relaxed, as you want them to be... and let that same relaxation spread down to the rest of your face, the cheeks, mouth and jaw muscles... that's right, that's good... it's a good feeling when you can notice those face muscles actually beginning to relax as much as they can, when you can feel the skin and the muscles of your face settling and smoothing out.

*"And, of course, you **can** feel those muscles settling as you relax them, because in your mind and brain, you have a mental map of your entire body... a mental map of your entire physical being... and that mental map is being checked **every single split second** of every day of your life by the automatic processes of your subconscious mind... and the odd thing is that you simply don't notice this happening... but you can also check any part of it with your conscious mind... so you can, if you wish, direct your thoughts to the very tip of the little finger on your right hand, for instance, and find it in your mind... there, you have it in your mind now... and you can see if you are able to think of **all** your finger tips at once... and even try to relax your fingertips as you think of them... and then you can direct your mind to, perhaps, your left knee... or your nose... or your right ear... and find those parts in your mind... and the odd thing is that you can be so unaware of other parts while you're testing those parts... so that until I finish this sentence, you probably won't have been aware of the sensations in the soles of your feet... but now you **are** aware of the sensations in the soles of your feet... but in becoming so, you've probably forgotten all about the tips of your fingers, even though they may still be relaxing...*

*"And it's a distinct oddity that that mental map is not as well detailed all over as you might imagine... so that, although you can locate, in your mind, the big toe on either foot... and the little toe on either foot... and **know** that you've located those parts of your body with total accuracy... if you try to think of the three toes between the little toe and the big toe... you begin to realise... that it feels for all the world as if there is only one more toe there... it just feels as though you have only a big toe, and a little toe, and only one toe in between... even though you consciously **know** there are three toes in between... and I wonder how many times in life there are contradic-*

*tions between something you can feel and something you know is different... or between something you believe and something that you **don't** realise is different... and as you ponder on these thoughts for just a moment or two... maybe continuing to check that mental map... seeing if you can relax every place you can think of... even relaxing your skin... even relaxing your bones... as you test the powers of your mind to access the tiniest parts of your body and relax them... I'd like you just to continue to listen quietly to the sound of my voice... and if your mind wanders quite a bit so that my voice just fades into the background, that's fine... and if it doesn't, that's fine too..."*

You will find that many people are ready to begin work at this point, though you can 'slide' into a suitable deepener quite unobtrusively at this point, especially if you use something like:

"... And I wonder if you can imagine how it would feel to explore that mental map... if you were standing on the terrace of a wonderful old building, like a stately home or a country mansion..."

The intuitive adaptable type

This personality is generally obliging and will tend to go along with whatever you ask him to do, within reason. His best response will almost always be to progressive relaxation—which he *loves*—and to any deepener which has soft imagery. Aim for the vocal equivalent of soft pastel colours. This brief relaxation routine, while not at all original, works extremely well and takes only two-and-a-half to three minutes to deliver. You can then use just about any deepener you wish, though many individuals will be in a deep enough working state by this time.

Relaxation

"Now I'd like you to think about the very top of your head... many people don't realise that tension often starts in the little muscles of the scalp, so I want you to think about those little muscles and the skin of your scalp and just allow them to let go and relax... now all the muscles of your face, just let them let go slack... your forehead and your eyes and eyelids... the cheeks, mouth and jaw muscles... it's a wonderful feeling when you let your face totally relax, because

you can actually feel the skin settling, smoothing out… it might mean that your mouth opens slightly, but whatever's best for you, just let it happen… unclenching your teeth and relaxing your tongue, because the more you physically relax, the more you can mentally relax… thinking about your neck and shoulder muscles now, and into the tops of your arms, letting all tensions drain away as you think on down through your elbows… into your forearms… down through your wrists and into your hands… right the way down into the very tips of your fingers and tips of your thumbs… just letting all those muscles let go and relax… and now think about your breathing, noticing that you're breathing even more steadily, even more slowly, as you relax more and more, so you can let any tension in the chest area simply drain away as you think on down to your stomach muscles, letting those muscles relax, too… think down into your back now, the long muscles either side of the spine, just let those muscles relax… and your waist… and your main thigh muscles, as you think on down through your knees, down through your shins and calves, just allowing all those areas to relax and let go, as you think on down through your ankles, through your feet, into the very tips of your toes… all the muscles of your body beautifully relaxed and easy… very lazy…"

Now you can move straight into any deepener if you feel it is necessary.

The charismatic evidential type

There is a low boredom threshold and a subsequent short concentration span often quite evident in this type of personality, so any induction needs to be novel and dynamic. The one shown here works extremely well, since the concept is novel enough to capture and hold the imagination, as well as focusing concentration upon breathing.

Handbreathing induction

"Now I'm going to ask you to concentrate on your breathing for a few moments… but I wonder if you can imagine a very strange idea… a very strange idea indeed… I wonder if you can imagine that you can actually breathe… through your fingertips… just imagine that rather strange idea that your fingers are just like hollow tubes…

that you can actually breathe in through the ends of those tubes... imagine that you can feel the air moving into your hands... quite slowly at first... just with a faint tingling sensation which you might feel on the back of your hands... or perhaps in your palms... and then just imagine that feeling moving slowly along your arms... through your elbows... just imagine that comforting flow of air moving through your elbows into your upper arms... and then into your shoulders... both arms... both shoulders... maybe finding again that faint tingling sensation... perhaps in your elbows or forearms this time... then moving down through the body... down into your legs... and through the main thigh muscles... through the knees into your shins and calves... and again, you might feel that faint tingling sensation, just there, just below your knees... then down through your ankles and into your feet... and out through your feet...

"And you can find a great deal of calmness and easiness... in that rather strange idea that you can breathe in through your fingers... that you can actually feel the air moving through your whole body... in one single, warming, comforting... unidirectional flow... and because it is a unidirectional flow of air.... moving through your whole body in one single comforting flow... the calmness and relaxation you breathe in... simply doesn't get involved with the tensions and stresses that you breathe away from yourself... the calmness and relaxation that you breathe in... simply doesn't get involved with the tensions and anxieties that you breathe away from yourself... so that with each breath you take... with each word I speak... you find yourself becoming steadily more and more... relaxed... with each breath you take, with each word I speak... you become steadily more and more... relaxed... beginning now, perhaps, to notice the weight of your head against the back of the chair... wondering if that weight might seem to gently increase as you relax even more... the weight of your feet on the footrest... wondering if that weight, too, might seem to gently increase... and some people can find that sensation of total relaxation... that feels as if they are actually beginning to sink gently through the chair... actually beginning to sink gently through the chair... so that it seems almost as if the chair is beginning to envelop you... you are so relaxed... a good feeling... a good feeling of calmness and safety... a safe calmness... that increases with each breath you take, with each word I speak... as you continue to breathe in through your fingers... allowing that comforting,

warming, relaxing flow of air... to move through your whole body and out through your feet...

"And this is something you can do for yourself whenever you want to... simply settle yourself into a comfortable position... with your eyes closed... then simply imagine yourself breathing in through your fingers.... imagine that flow of air comforting and relaxing every part of your body.... then breathing out through your feet... and each time you breathe out just say to yourself: 'Relax... now...'... just saying: 'Relax... now...' to yourself with each breath you breathe... and saying: 'Relax... now...' will act as a trigger to your subconscious mind... and on the fourth time you say it... on the fourth time you say it... you'll find yourself to be more relaxed... than you've ever been before..."

You may wish to follow this routine with a deepener, and if you do, make quite certain that it has a lot of powerful imagery in which your client can easily involve his mind. The passive type of deepener that you might use for the IA personality type, with relaxing imagery like lakes, streams, mountains and so on can actually be boring to the CE type and will not necessarily deepen the state of hypnosis. A trip round a vividly created fairground or an imaginary journey through his own body would be far better. With the right client, a motorcycle race around Brand's Hatch would be even better!

Part Two

Analytical Work

Chapter 9

Techniques for Regression and Analysis

The object of regression or analytical work is to discover the underlying cause of an individual's symptom pattern and satisfactorily resolve the associated conflicts. There are two distinctly separate, though related, methods of achieving this that may be employed:

(1) Regression to cause, which seeks to follow a memory path down to the first time the symptom pattern or associated emotional response was experienced during the *initial sensitising event (ISE)*. The conflicts generated may then be worked through so that negative emotions may be released.

(2) Free association, the Freudian method of analysis. Here, the object of the exercise is the same, but the route is far less direct, taking in a wider area of your client's life and usually concentrating on childhood.

Each system has its own particular strengths and weaknesses and the professional therapist should be familiar and confident with both, and easily able to decide which is better for any individual client. We will have a look at an overview of each before going into details of methodology.

Regression to cause

This is indicated particularly with the client who is able to function quite normally and satisfactorily except in one area of life. The sufferer from a fear/phobia or other reactive state who remains perfectly comfortable as long as she is able to avoid her specific trigger situation is a typical candidate. Fear of flying, specific social fears, claustrophobia and agoraphobia, anxiety about authority figures—anything where the symptom is predominantly of an emotional/psychological nature—all 'qualify' here. Regression to cause can also be used where there is a physical illness that may have a psychological cause—again, we are looking at a single specific symptom.

The advantages of this particular method are that the client is usually aware from the very beginning of therapy that progress is being made; it can often be very fast, satisfying today's requirement for brief therapy; and it is easy to explain to your client what you are going to do and why you are going to do it. Because of its more interactive (between therapist and client) nature, it can achieve results where free association might fail.

The disadvantage is that it follows a relatively narrow path to the originating cause and this can leave important areas of emotional development unexplored. As a result there may be conflict(s) which may not be resolved, and unreleased repressions which may be triggered at a later date, producing a whole new symptom pattern. Also, it is unlikely to work effectively where there are multiple symptoms.

Free association

A typical analysis using free association in the way that Freud taught had a duration of a thousand hours—that is three sessions a week for seven years! Fortunately, combining free association with hypnosis shortens this more than somewhat, so that a successful outcome can often be achieved within only six or so sessions, making for a truly brief therapy. Even where the difficulties are great, a 'long' therapy in this context is still only a matter of months, not years. This is because bypassing the conscious critical faculty through the judicious use of a suitable induction, allows 'secret' thoughts to surface far more readily than when using the consciously coercive method that is often employed by the 'standard' psycho-analyst.

The use of this method is indicated when your client presents to you with multiple symptoms which tend to affect most parts of her life; there is often general anxiety, low self-esteem, low self-confidence, possibly panic attacks (random and triggered) and/or psychosexual difficulty, low libido, etc., *in addition* to her main presenting symptom which may very well be a phobia or fear of some sort. She may not even be fully aware that she actually suffers some of the other problems until you start to gather information about the way she is and how she functions. Quite often, she supposes that severe low self-esteem, for example, is something she will always have to put up with and will express disbelief that she could ever feel much different. "It's just the way I am," is a very common statement and the reason for that is simple: *You cannot know how you would be if you were not as you are.*

This method really comes into its own—has no equal, in fact—when it comes to dealing with what used to be called 'hysterical illness'. Here, there is almost always a *physical* symptom evident: nausea/vomiting, black-outs or fainting fits, psoriasis, eczema and other skin conditions, attacks of blindness, sleeping problems, paralysis of part or even all of the body, all of the various forms of impotence (including inhibited or premature ejaculation), anorgasmia and vaginismus… to name but a few.

The advantages of using free association are that it is not necessary for your client to follow a specific train of thought (in fact, there will quite often be three or four in evidence at any one time); thus she will 'clear up' all sorts of unfinished childhood business during her therapy in addition to resolving her main symptom, and so reduce the potential to become psychologically ill again; and there is a 'side effect' of increased self-confidence and generally lowered stress levels.

The disadvantages are that it can be slower than direct regression, even though it often is not; also, it is not uncommon for it to seem as if nothing at all is happening as a result of the therapy until at least session five—when it happens in a rush; and the client's mood can be extremely variable during the period that she is in therapy.

Although free association is a separate therapy model, much of the technique can be, and often is, used in a limited manner during direct regression-to-cause therapy.

In practice

And so we come to the details of the methodologies as they are employed by the professional therapist in the consulting room. The theory behind them is not covered here, merely the method by which we work.

We will begin with the regression-to-cause model. There are various forms of this, but they are mostly based on the *Watkins Affect Bridge* technique, which has been in use for some considerable time now. There are certain things which are common to both therapy models, and they are covered in a later part of the chapter.

Before the induction, ascertain when your client last experienced the symptom pattern—ideally this will have been within the few days prior to the session. After you have conducted whatever induction/deepener you feel is appropriate, continue with something like:

> *"All right (name), now I'd like you to focus on that feeling that we talked about a few minutes ago… and what I want you to do is to use all your imagination to make that as absolutely vivid as you can, while I count from one to five… make it as vivid and as real in your mind as you can possibly stand it to be…"*

Count 1–5 slowly. Increase excitation whilst watching for signs of unease (it needs to be there) urging on the client and slowing the count down if necessary. A bio-feedback meter helps enormously, here. The hypnotic state will usually increase quite dramatically. Then:

> *"Good! That's excellent! Now just stay focused on that feeling in your mind while I count from ten to one… your mind might want to go to thoughts but make sure you stay focused on just that **feeling**… and as I count from ten back to one, your subconscious is going to look back through time, all the way back through time, to a memory or a person or a place or maybe just a thought from way back, that has absolutely everything to do with that **feeling** and when I get to one I want you to tell me the very first thing that pops into your mind."*

Now count from ten down to one, slowly, allowing a considerable pause between 'two' and 'one'.

Most of the time, at the count one, your client will tell you something she remembers from the past and you work with it, exploring it until it's exhausted. Here is an example of the sort of thing you might find:

Client: I'm remembering being in the school playground…

Therapist: (say nothing if it's not absolutely necessary to speak)

Client: It's my first day at school… I don't like it…

Therapist: And you don't like that first day at school, because…?

Client: Because I feel frightened.

Therapist: You feel frightened… and what happens then?

Client: (uncomfortable) My mum leaves me. (little tears)

Therapist:

… more school memories …

Some minutes later:

Client: I'm still in the classroom…but I'm older now…

Therapist: And what's happening in that classroom while you're older?

Client: (little draw of breath) The teacher's shouting!

Therapist:

Client: Someone's been naughty… not me, though. Somebody else has been naughty. The teacher's shouting and his face is all red!

Shift of attention

Now here is a change—the attention has shifted from the client on to somebody else. But the concept is important since it involves emotion, as well as guilt and punishment (naughty child, shouting teacher). You could pursue this further if there was sufficient client emotion evident to indicate that it was directly relevant, otherwise we could proceed thus:

"Good, okay, now I want you to focus on that teacher's shouting and his red face... really focus on how that feels and make it as vivid as you can while I count from one to five...and if your mind jumps somewhere else, that's fine, you can focus on that instead, and if it doesn't, that's fine, too."

Now repeat the process as shown above. And that's all there is to it, really... except that you need to be constantly alert to keep your client orientated to self and to watch for when the train of thought is becoming exhausted or diverted in some way. Then you would choose the last point at which there was emotion present—it doesn't matter *which* emotion—and focus your client onto that before starting the process again.

It's not always necessary to do the counting once you've got your client started—especially if she is a good client. When the train of thought wavers, refocus your client's attention on the last emotional point, then tell her to just simply let her mind drift for a moment and tell you the next thing she thinks of. Then continue with the process as before. This technique is 'borrowed' from free association methodology.

Sometimes a train of thought will last for only a few minutes, while at other times it could last an entire session. Although it is unlikely to happen in just one session (though sometimes it does), your client will sooner or later home in on that initial sensitising event.

There are two things which will make it obvious that it *is* the originating cause of your client's problems. One is the amount of emotion that is generated during the recall—although, in reality, it is being released, rather than generated. There will also quite often be physical responses evident in the form of motor action.

The second is that after you have 'worked through' the event, your client will be able to review it with a great deal less emotional response and may even profess to feel nothing at all other than a sense of euphoria or elation. Later, in the section concerned with Common Factors, you will read of a third circumstance which makes it even more obvious that you have released the originating cause.

An alternative

You have read and understood (hopefully!) what should happen, in the normal way. Sometimes, though, resistance kicks in and what you actually get after counting down from ten to one, is: "Nothing, sorry, nothing at all..."

No problem! Just ask the client to answer the questions you ask her with the first thing that comes into her mind. What might follow is something like:

Therapist: Okay, just give me your first impressions now... is it light or dark?

Client: Light...

Therapist: Ok, and are you indoors or outdoors when it's light?

Client: Indoors...

Therapist: Good. And are you alone or are you with other people when you're indoors and it's light?

Client: My Mum's there.

Therapist: Good. Your Mum's there. And how old are you when your Mum's there and you're indoors and it's light?

Client: I'm seven.

Therapist: You're seven. And what else is there about that when you're seven and your Mum's there and you're indoors and it's light...?

You get the idea. Build up and feed back what the client has told you. There are many other things you can ask, always feeding back as much of the information that your client has given you as you sensibly can. It's important that you must never actually *lead* your clients, only *guide* them—there's more about leading and guiding in Chapter Ten, but for now it's sufficient to understand that you should say nothing which carries a suggestion embedded within it.

For instance: "Who else is there with you?" **leads** your client, while: "And are you on your own?" does not. But: "And are you all on your own?" is emotive (because of the connotations of vulnerability in 'all on your own') and leads your client into a possibly erroneous reaction which may belong to an entirely different memory altogether. "Didn't that feel awful?" is a blatant lead, but: "How did that feel to you?" is perfectly all right. Yes, you are quite right, it *is* difficult... but remember, it's *only* difficult...

The following are useful and safe (not in any particular order):

"What clothes are you wearing?"

"Are you hot or cold or just comfortable?"

"Is it sunny or cloudy?"

"Are you happy or sad or 'just there'?"

"How does Mum (or whoever) look?"

"Where could you be going?"

"Where could you be?"

"What could you be doing?"

"What could be happening there?"

"Where could Mum (or whoever) be?" (when 'my mum's not there' has been volunteered)

"I wonder when that could have been?"

"I wonder how old you could be?"

It is a good idea to list as many such questions as you can think of, checking that they are only guides, of course. Notice that they are all questions—observations must be used sparingly and with extreme caution; any observational work is going to be a result of your own thought processes, which may not suit the client at all.

Once you get her going, it is not usually too long before your client will say something along the lines of: "Oh, I remember now, this was the time when…" Then, of course, you work with it and explore it as necessary.

À la Freud

Now we come to free association—the invention of that often unfairly criticised pioneer of psychotherapy, Sigmund Freud. Yes, some of his ideas are bizarre, old-fashioned, sexist, and do not hold water at all; but many of them are as sound today as they were when he propounded them. Free association is one of those.

We seek the same end result as with direct regression work, hopefully releasing a repressed memory (which might be purely an emotion), allowing our client to let go of the psychological burden that has beset her. The major difference with this method is that it is far less interactive and direct. The therapist's major contribution at the beginning is to teach the client how to free-associate in the first place, to encourage her in her early efforts, and to watch for resistance and attempts to evade issues (more about that later in this chapter), gently leading her back on course if necessary.

The main problem with this method, though, is that it is just too easy! In fact, it is so easy that it can sometimes be difficult unless you use your personality and charisma to convince the client that she is actually doing the right thing.

Free association simply means allowing the subconscious mind to make links between ideas and concepts with as little interference as possible from conscious thought processes. Once in hypnosis, we ask our client to cast her mind back to her earliest years (we work almost exclusively in the childhood years during free association) and tell us the first thing she thinks of, without analysing it, without questioning it in any way. Then, without trying to make any connection at all in the conscious mind, tell us the next thing that comes to mind. Then the next… and the next, and so on. As simple as that. Well, very nearly; we need to make sure that what we teach our client to do is to tell us not simply memories, but psychological experiences.

The difference between a memory and a psychological experience is that the former may well be just of the physical details of an event, whilst the latter will employ the emotional responses as well. The majority of people will do this automatically but some, especially those who have been subject to repeated abuse (not necessarily sexual), will seek to avoid confronting those emotional states. You will have to work a little harder with those individuals, maybe asking them to go back over something that seems as if there should be more of an emotional response than is apparent, and getting them to imagine that they are there right now, right this minute.

After one or two sessions of your reminding your client what you want her to do, you should find that she will be silent for no more than a few seconds between recalls—indeed she **must not** be silent for more than a few seconds, for this would mean she was being selective in relating her thoughts—the exact opposite of what is supposed to happen! We want the very first thought each time, if our work is to be effective.

The subconscious thought processes will unerringly move towards 'unfinished business' from those formative years—and that is where the origins of hysterical illness are to be found. It doesn't matter too much that you may not yet fully understand why this should be so—just happily accept, for the moment, that it is!

It will be every bit as obvious as it is in direct regression, and in the same way, when you have touched on matters of importance; but there is a major difference in that with this method you can quite easily find that the first major emotional release you discover is the originating cause of your client's symptoms.

The setting up of your client is somewhat different, too, for this method. On each session, after a suitable induction and deepener, you could use the first paragraph of the script in Chapter Five, or anything similar that served as a reminder of childhood. Follow that with: *"And now I want you to gather up a memory, and I want you to tell me the very first thing, the very first thing, that comes up into your conscious mind."*

Whereas in direct regression work the therapist will be almost constantly interacting with the client, the reverse is more the case here. All the time your client is doing her job properly, i.e. constantly relating a series of psychological experiences to you, you should remain as 'invisible' as possible—no comments, no rationalisation, no interference. Let your client find her own way through it; this does not mean that all you have to do is sit quietly and just let your client get on with it. On the odd occasion that you get the perfect client, that may very well be the case, but with the others, there are certain things to watch for besides unadmitted emotion, certain things to bear in mind and correct if necessary. These are:

(1) Recalls need to be of actual events, rather than vague descriptions of the way things used to be, such as the client's daily journey to school, aimless wandering in the mind around the area where she lived, etc. The 'slide show' technique in Chapter Seventeen is an excellent aid for this.

(2) Sequential or chronological recalls are not free association and won't get your client to where she wants to be. Example: "I remember a holiday... we're getting into the car... now we're driving along the road... now we're stopping for a picnic... but Dad wants us to get going again..." and so on.

(3) Diversions along the lines of: "I thought this was where I lived when I was five but now I'm not certain, because I can remember a tree in the garden and we didn't have a tree in the garden of that house, so I'm not sure..."

(4) Not admitting a memory. A bio-feedback meter will reveal this by a sudden sharp increase in the reading. Body language will often show it, too, in sudden 'waggling' movements of the feet (an

urge to run away) or in other sudden movements, especially turning the head away from you.

(5) Deletion. This is shown by disconnected statements like: "My father was a good man." Why has she said that? Is she justifying something? Something is missing, deleted. Maybe there should be a "but…" at the end of that statement! Sometimes it can be this sort of thing: "I'd have loved to have piano lessons…" So why didn't she? Something missing again. The therapist needs to explore these areas. A good way to do this is to rephrase the statement if necessary and put a question at the end of it: "And you didn't have piano lessons, because…?" Always use 'because?' rather than 'why?'—it begs a far more direct answer.

As you may be beginning to realise, free association can be a more difficult discipline than direct regression, but it is one well worth learning, and an extremely powerful healing tool.

Case study

Here's a tiny fragment of an actual case.

Client: I'm remembering being in a race on school sports day.

Therapist:

Client: I didn't want to run in it…

Therapist: Because…?

Client: Billy Brown was in it and he'd hit me if I beat him. He was a bully.

Therapist: (getting client to resume) And you're in that race. And what happened then?

Client: I came second. (sigh) I always came second at everything.

Therapist:

Client: I never won anything. I always felt so useless.

Therapist:

Client: My little sister always used to win things... (grimace)

Therapist:

Client: My little sister was Dad's favourite. It's not fair. (little tears)

Therapist:

Client: It's still the same, even now... (Resistance! The client's mind has turned away from childhood feelings of inadequacy and hurt.)

Therapist: Now let your mind drop right back to those childhood years and tell me the very first thing you think of.

Five minutes later, the client was vividly remembering the feelings of hopelessness and despair when her father repeatedly insisted that her young sister was far brighter than she was and that she would never be as successful. It was the beginning of a release of cumulative trauma which had produced severe 'weekend migraine' symptoms from the age of eighteen onwards, when she had left school and started work. Of course, it was at weekends that she had most contact with her father; the migraine symptom served the purpose of her having to lie down in a darkened, quiet room, thus escaping the constant harangue and the proof that she was inadequate and maybe unlovable. The subconscious had continued the symptom even after she had left home.

The case dialogue clearly shows how free association works. The subconscious thought processes homed in on a competitive situation, then bullying, feelings of inadequacy, injustice, and finally hopelessness.

Common factors

Now we come to some common ground, elements that are equally important in both methods of analysis. One has already been touched upon, that of GUIDING and not LEADING. This is written in capital letters because it is of **enormous importance** that you thoroughly learn the difference between the two before you ever begin to conduct this sort of work. Any **leading** could distort the end result of therapy to the point where your client would have been infinitely better off if she had never consulted with you in the first place.

Getting this wrong will damage your client, your reputation, your bank balance, and the hypnotherapy profession as a whole. It is covered in greater detail in Chapter Ten.

Repression

Sometimes a client will recall an event or circumstance that seems to her as if it is something completely new. She knows beyond doubt that it *is* a memory, but it seems to her it had somehow lain hidden in some dark recess in her mind since the day it happened. This is what is known as a *repressed memory*. Repression theory is not covered in this book, but just accept the repressed memory as something which has been out of sight of your client's conscious mind until this very moment. The obvious release of a repression is proof positive that you have hit the originating cause of symptoms. It is accompanied by *abreaction* (covered later in this chapter).

At this moment, there is usually an understanding for both therapist and client as to why and how those particular symptoms were 'chosen' by the subconscious mind as a reaction set.

When it is released, the emotional processes which created the repression can no longer have an effect upon your client's psyche—it is no longer a secret and therefore there is nothing to hide, nothing for the subconscious to engineer avoidance for. That avoidance was the reason for the symptom pattern in the first place, and it is not an exaggeration to say that the curative effects upon your client can be truly astounding. The one-time sufferer of claustrophobia no longer notices whether or not she is in a small space; the former agoraphobia sufferer now *loves* walking through the park or on the beach; the shy social recluse now adores parties.

Of course, the client is absolutely astonished by this; not that she's remembered the event... but that she ever forgot it in the first place! She will often say: "I think I knew about that all the time, really. I just didn't want to face it." And of course, there is an element of truth there. But the most fascinating thing is when she says: "You know, I don't really think it was all that bad, really..." or: "I don't think we actually found very much, did we?" This last is usually after releasing a trauma that would send even the strongest amongst us quivering into a corner!

On occasions, this classic line comes up: "Oh, yes, I feel so much better now, thanks. No disrespect to you, but I don't think it had much to do with the hypnosis—I think I must've been about to get better anyway..." Now, at that point, the professional therapist simply smiles, wishes the client a good life, and sends her on her way... content in the knowledge that they have done their job well enough that the client is now a totally independent individual, just as she was designed to be.

Our job as therapists is not to get gratitude and ego-stroking from our clients. They come to us for help and if we do the job properly they should totally forget about us afterwards. How many times do you think about your dentist if your teeth don't ache? If this seems not to sit too well with you, if you feel that your clients should be eternally grateful for your help in sorting out their life... then closely examine your motives for wanting to be a therapist in the first place. The successful therapist cares sufficiently about a client that the most important thing is to help her to function as 'normally' as if her problems had never existed, as if she had never had to visit the therapist's office in the first place.

Abreaction

An abreaction—the revivication of a traumatic experience from the past—always accompanies the release of repression; it is as if the mind/body still has to discharge whatever was motivated at the time, even though that time is now long gone. Tears still flow, anger still shouts, fists might still flail and fear can drive feet to want to run. In other words, an abreaction can include physical motor action as well as emotions.

There are three possible experiences in an abreactive state which can be felt singly or simultaneously:

(1) The event itself—as a visual/auditory experience. It is almost inevitably accompanied by either or both of the other two experiences below.

(2) The physical (kinaesthetic) sensations—touch, pain, or other tactile sensations. *Anything* may be experienced, even orgasm (though it should be borne in mind that most repressions are created at a quite early age), hence the motor action that is observed from time to time. Physical sensations may be felt without the experience of the event itself.

(3) The emotional response—whatever feelings were present, which may frequently be guilt, albeit unwarranted. It is by no means unusual for emotions to be released with no conscious knowledge of the event that the emotion is connected to. This is by far the most common manifestation of abreaction.

Although abreaction can be quite dramatic, it certainly is not always so; depending upon personality type, it can be anything from a silent tear or two up to thrashing of arms and legs accompanied by blood-curdling shrieks! Abreacted emotion is the 'trademark' of success of any form of hypnoanalysis; it is the important part of the work, for it is an essential occurrence if our clients are to be healed.

There is often a need to 'work through' the trauma that has been brought into consciousness in this way and, again, the 'slide show' technique in Chapter Seventeen is an admirable aid for this.

Be very certain in your mind that you have mastered at least one technique for working through trauma before beginning any type of analytical or regression therapy with a client.

Session resistance

This can take several forms, one being a tendency to analyse and rationalise every memory; the client tells you something and follows it with: "I suppose that's why I've always..." etc. or: "I wonder why I've thought of that?" This type of resistive response will severely inhibit therapy and must be instantly discouraged. Insist that the client just tells you what she is thinking and then moves on to the next memory/thought, without trying to work out any reasons or rationale. A slightly jokey: "Now, you just do the remembering and I'll do the analysing!" usually does the trick.

Another form of resistance is the 'blank'—the: "I'm sorry, I just can't seem to think of anything…" response. Since it is a near-impossibility to completely empty your mind without several years of training in meditative techniques, this is unlikely to truly be the case. There is always a thought there somewhere but it may be either a shameful thought she does not want to tell you about, something that she has judged to be unimportant, not what you are waiting for, not the cause of her problems… or any one of dozens of rationales to avoid telling you what is in her mind.

It should be made quite clear to your client from the outset that she must tell you absolutely everything that comes to mind. It is a good idea to tell her that the four golden rules are:

(1)   Nothing is too shameful and therefore censored.

(2)   Nothing is too trivial.

(3)   No thought is irrelevant.

(4)   NO SECRETS!

It is when encountering any of the many and various forms of session resistance that the best therapists are separated from the also-rans. The good ones simply do not quit! They *insist* on the client doing her part of the work and use anything they can to get the client relating her thoughts as they come to her, without checking everything through first to ensure that it is safe. The therapist's determination to get the client through a good therapy will be obvious to the client and will go a long way towards dispelling any resistance that may rear its head.

In general, if it becomes obvious that your client is holding back and not telling you everything and you cannot get her to do so by about session four, then you need to be insistent that she **must** start to do her part of the work or you will have to terminate her sessions with you. This might be seen as quitting by some; to others, keeping that client in therapy could be seen as opportunism and motivated by financial gain, since she is unlikely to improve in her emotional wellbeing. Look after your clients properly, guard your reputation well, and your appointment book will always be full.

While this chapter contains a fairly comprehensive overview of analytical and regression methods, it is not intended as a complete methodology, but as a starting point for those not already familiar with this work. The very best of therapists are in a continuous learning process and this is even more important for the therapist engaged in any form of 'uncovering' work.

There are many courses and seminars available to therapists wishing to improve their knowledge, and browsing through the catalogues of specialist book suppliers will also turn up works related to regression and analysis. Although he is considered out of date, you would do well to study some of Freud's writing in the subject; he was the pioneer, and much of what he wrote still stands any therapist in good stead.

Chapter 10

Rapid Cognitive Linguistics

What you say to your client, especially during an analytical/ regression session, is no more and no less important than what you don't say! Saying the wrong thing (or saying the right thing but saying it wrongly) can imply all sorts of other meanings, and you should be very aware that your client is in an extraordinarily suggestible state when you are talking to him, even if he has only just arrived in your office and has yet to enter the state of hypnosis.

This chapter is all about guiding and leading and the importance of using one and conscientiously avoiding the other at all costs. **Guiding** means encouraging your client to think along the right lines as far as you can perceive them in an attempt to bring him to a truth. **Leading** is suggesting to the client in some way that he has experienced a sensation or event that you believe would account for his symptom(s). **Guiding** helps to uncover the client's truth; **Leading** implants the therapist's idea of a possible truth—*which will at best partially alleviate the client's symptom(s) for no more than a short while, at worst positively* **guarantee** *that the client will* **never** *be able to find the relief he seeks.*

Your clients believe that you are knowledgeable and aware of things which they know nothing about, and, of course, they are right; they would not be coming to you for treatment if this were not the case. They know you are an 'expert' at understanding human behaviour and they believe that you already have some idea of what is wrong with them and why they have their particular set of symptoms. Therefore, if you suggest, albeit only by implication, that there may be something more to what they are telling you, then they will make strenuous efforts to find it… all well and good, except for the fact that they will be sure to find *something* even if there is, in reality, nothing to find.

Be careful what you look for

If you find yourself doubting that fact, just remember that the human mind has a predisposition to keep on looking for what it expects to discover. If we are looking for evidence that somebody does not like us, for example—probably out of fear that we might find it—we will not be content with two or three or even ten instances that seem to show the opposite. We will keep on looking for that *one* piece of evidence that we are searching for until we find it—or something else that can be easily misconstrued as 'proof'. And then that belief system has been reinforced and the knowledge that you are not liked has been confirmed. This famous saying is certainly true:

"Be very careful what you look for, because you'll find it."

Consider the following.

The client says:

"I remember Dad coming into my room."

The therapist might say any of these:

"And what did he do, after he came into the room?"

"Aha! Did he, indeed!"

"Did he often come into your room?"

"And were you frightened?"

"Oh no! I bet that scared you!"

"How did that seem to you?"

Any of those statements/questions could and probably would lead the client into searching for some unpleasant, even sinister, reason for Dad having come into the room. We'll look at them in order, but first we will assume that Dad actually did nothing more than say 'Goodnight' before turning out the light and leaving.

Implications

"And what did he do, after he came into the room?" This implies that Dad did, indeed, do something. Some clients—more than you might imagine—would actually find themselves complying with that unspoken suggestion and claiming that Dad actually *did* do something. It might be something quite innocent, but the therapist who leads would soon be sowing doubts all over the place about whether or not Dad always behaved as Dads should.

"Aha! Did he indeed!" There is massive implication here that something is definitely amiss, that this absolutely must mean something. This is especially true if the client has been educated about repression and 'buried' memories. Now remember that famous statement quoted above.

"Did he often come into your room?" The implication here should not need pointing out! It suggests that he may well have done and poses the question 'Why?' The therapist's interest in this indicates that this is possibly abnormal and should be investigated.

"And were you frightened?" Suggests the client should have been, or that it would not be unusual to be so.

"Oh no! I bet that scared you!" Similar to above, but far more blatant.

"How did that seem to you?" Depending on the tone of voice used, this can suggest that there should have been a specific feeling about the event, rather than a feeling of normality. Some clients would smile and answer: *"Nice…"*. But others, who may not have enjoyed an especially good relationship with their father, might begin to wonder exactly how they *did* feel, and that, along with other implications relayed by the therapist, could lead into very stormy waters indeed.

The point is, any of those responses listed above could lead to unwitting confabulation by the client, and further leading and collusion by the therapist might very well exacerbate the situation to the point where there is a real possibility of a false memory/belief being generated.

For what it's worth, we (the authors) don't believe that false memory actually exists, as such. The perception of an event, and the storing of such, is a function of the physical **brain**; memory and interpretation of memory is a function of the non-physical **mind**. This chapter is not about false memory, so we won't go too deeply into it here, but suffice it to say for the moment that a *false belief* is a very different matter and certainly entirely possible. Think about it until you understand that memory and belief are not the same thing at all.

The best response

So what *should* the therapist have responded with? Easy!

Nothing at all.

Saying nothing would have been the best response, here. The client's mind was already likely to remember anything that *had* happened without further prompting. Now, if for any reason the therapist decided that there was a need to investigate this event further—the client remaining silent for too long, for example, or grimacing, or perhaps suddenly shuffling his feet (a very useful body language signal indicating discomfort of some sort)—then it would be in order to carefully explore the situation.

"And what happened then?" delivered in a calm and measured tone is a safe response that can be used frequently; it implies nothing specific and merely asks for the next thing that happened. As a matter of interest, asking: *"And what happened **next**?"* will tend to produce a slightly different response, in that the client will be likely to remember the next event, rather than the next part of the existing event.

There is a system of what is often referred to as 'effective reflective language' invented by the English therapist, David Grove, that is very useful, too. Here, you would feed back what the client has just said, then prompt for the next response. Something like: *"And you remember Dad coming into your room… And what happened then…?"* This principle can be followed, building up until we are feeding back three or four 'elements' of the situation that our client has given us.

We then get something like: *"And Dad comes into your room… and you're lying in bed… and he turns the light on… and stands inside the door…and when he's stood there long enough…what happens then?"*

There is more about this method, along with a list of some suitable responses in Chapter Nine. It's a slow process—but we're going for long-term cures here, not speed. In any case, you'd only need to use it when your client's recall seems to be faltering.

The 'awkward' client

In truth, there is no such thing as an awkward client… but some of them certainly *seem* like they are! Silences, blanks, reiterations, reminiscences, refusals, justifications, deletions, downright lies… these are just some of the situations that can easily frustrate the unwary therapist into asking leading questions. The various ways of dealing with these situations are covered elsewhere; in this chapter we are going to keep firmly to the subject of guiding, rather than leading.

In general, it is safer to ask questions than to make observations, unless that observation is made in a dissociated manner, such as: *"Of course, sometimes it's possible to feel an emotional response that seems to come out of nowhere…"* as opposed to: *"I think it's possible that you might feel…"* etc. But any questions you ask must be totally free from suggestion.

There were some examples of suggestive questions earlier in this chapter all relating to a specific circumstance. Here are some more, one or two of which it is only too easy to find yourself asking. Each one of them carries a specific implication; work out what it is and think how you could ask each without leading.

"Who else is there with you?"

"Did that feel nice or nasty?"

"Is s/he making you touch her/him?"

"What else did s/he do/say?"

"How many times did that happen?"

"Did s/he/you do a bad thing?"

"When did you see him/her again?"

"Did s/he ever come into your room?"

"Did you see things you should not have seen?"

As a matter of interest, if you believe that there is a sexual connotation to some of these questions, then that is a perfect example of the hidden lead. There is actually no direct reference to anything sexual at all in any of them, and the only reason you might think that there is, is because of a tendency or predisposition to do so because of past conditioning. *Many, if not all, of your clients will be subject to those same conditioning processes.* Of course, it does depend, to an extent, on the context within which those questions are asked, but if you get into the habit of not leading just as soon as you possibly can, then you will always be 'safe', won't you?

By now, you should be beginning to get some 'feel' about what is okay and what is not okay. But we are not finished yet.

Impartiality

One of the most difficult things for the therapist to do is to remain totally non-judgemental and non-critical, and totally open-minded about the origins of our clients' symptom pattern—and yet we absolutely have to do that if we are to be truly successful. If you start to form an opinion about what event has befallen your client in the past, it won't be long before you fall into the 'be careful what you look for' trap. And you know what happens then!

As far as being non-judgemental and non-critical is concerned, well, that should not be difficult. We have all said and done things we should not have said or done, so none of us has the right to sit in judgement upon another. But it is the open-mindedness about the symptom(s) that is more difficult. So here is a piece of advice:

ALWAYS KEEP AN OPEN MIND.

Never underestimate the perceptiveness of the subconscious mind; if you think an idea strongly enough, then every action, every word, every tone and nuance of speech, everything about you will convey that idea to your client just as certainly as if you had written it in letters ten feet high!

You might say: *"And what else is there about that?"*—a perfectly valid 'clean' response. But if you privately thought that there was something untoward about 'that', then subtle voice tones could well be responsible for your client hearing: *"Aha! And what else is there about THAT then, eh?"* Obviously, you would not make it that apparent and you certainly would not be aware of those nuances yourself; but rest assured that the mere thought that there was something to find would ensure that it would be there. We should always let our client do most of the work, wherever possible—he alone knows what ails him and the cause of it, even if that knowledge is only at a subconscious level. If we do our job properly, those subconscious processes will become conscious memories that can be rationalised/desensitised and our client's problem will soon cease to be.

Case study

Here is a fragment of a genuine case that illustrates perfectly the need to let the client do most of the work. This was a young woman presenting with difficulties in the sexual area of relationships, unease with men generally, and low self-esteem. Hypnoanalysis and free association was the chosen method of therapy. The symbolism here is more than usually important and it would be a useful exercise to think what the therapist might have said that would have been injurious.

On session four, the young woman had been feeling uneasy for ten minutes or so, then:

> **Client:** *I'm in the shed playing with Daddy's stick. Daddy likes me playing with his stick.*

> **Therapist:** *What else is there about that?*

> **Client:** *Um… Daddy says not to tell mummy.*

Therapist:

Client: *I have to hold it a special way.*

Therapist:

Client: *Daddy gets cross if I don't hold it a special way... (big frown) He's showing me how to hold it.*

Therapist: *And what happens then?*

Client: *I don't know... he just gets cross, 'cos I won't hold it properly. (another frown) Something's not right here, though.*

Therapist: *(guiding) Something's not right here, because...?* ('Because?' is much better than 'why?', since it is more specific and therefore doesn't so easily allow justifications.)

Client: *When I hold it right... it's just too hard...*

Therapist: *What is it that's just too hard?*

Client: *(another frown) To hold it. Too heavy for me to hold it properly. (giggles) I told my mum!*

Therapist: *And what happened then?*

Client: *She told Daddy off... 'cos girls don't play cricket.*

Daddy's 'stick' turned out to be a cricket bat and my client was describing it with the vocabulary of the four-year-old she was remembering being! The 'symbolism' turned out to be nothing more than the semantics of a child. Now, of course, we could have really made something out of that apparent sexual content and the client might very well have taken our lead and either become carried away with the idea of abuse, or horrified that something of a sexual nature *had* indeed happened at some point. Either way, the therapy would have been hurt. We would have given her the idea that:

(1) There must be a sexual abuse at the root of her problems.

(2) The therapist was looking for sexual abuse and therefore she should, too.

(3) (Worst case) She had better stop therapy in case she discovers some form of sexual abuse.

In the event, her main problem was nothing more sinister than a cumulative trauma brought about by the fact that her father had desperately wanted a son. This resulted in years of his attempting to mould her into a tomboy, which had provoked a conflict between her feminine instincts and how she perceived (via Dad) she had to be if men were to like her.

There is another 'golden rule' of therapy also illustrated here. Always be absolutely certain that you know what your client is actually talking about before you *do anything with* what they're talking about. Ask questions, wait patiently, guide them back on path if they stray… but always wait until you know what they're talking about.

Guiding

Now we'll have a look at the process of guiding a client to any place that we feel he should be. But remember, we must always be prepared to accept that we might be wrong, that it is only *our* feeling that he needs to be there.

Guiding is simply persuading the client, as 'invisibly' as possible, to be more specific about a certain point or to have another or closer 'look' at something he's remembered. We would do this if we were absolutely certain, for some reason, that he was missing something or not making a connection.

We will use a hypothetical situation where the client has obviously been subject to some sort of trauma in the school playground (body language and/or bio-feedback equipment has told us there is stress associated) but appears to be 'turning away' from it.

>*Client: I don't like the playground. I'm going to think about the classroom.*

95

Therapist: What else is there about the playground? (Attempting to recreate the focus of attention to where it had been.)

Client: I'm remembering being in Miss Jones' class. She was nice, Miss Jones…I liked Miss Jones.

Therapist: Tell me about that. (Staying away from the playground momentarily to allow the client to regain confidence that he is 'in charge'.)

Client: She was always smiling… all the time.

Therapist: While she was teaching you?

Client: Yes… while she was teaching us.

Therapist: And when Miss Jones had finished teaching you… what happened then? (Blatant, but effective. When classes finish, then, at some point, the pupils must be back in the playground!)

Client: Don't remember…

Therapist: I wonder what happened then—when Miss Jones had finished teaching you?

Client: I don't want to go back into the playground…

Therapist: And you don't want to go back into the playground, because…?

It should be fairly straightforward from here.

Gently does it

You get the idea. Think logically and *gently* steer your client back to where he should go. It might take a few attempts, but all the time he is resisting, the more likely it is that there is a sound reason to get him to look there. After all, if there was not, there would be no resistance!

Another situation may be where a client is telling you about a situation or event where it is quite obvious that there *should* be some sort of emotion evident, but nothing is showing. There, we could say something like: *"All right, now be there in your mind, just as if it was happening right this very minute… and now tell me how that feels to you… how does that feel?"* which, if we do our job convincingly, should produce the emotional connection. If he starts to turn away from it, then we can do this sort of thing: *"Go on, go on… be there in your mind! Tell me how that feels… go on… it's safe, it's okay… give it room in your body and let yourself **feel** how that feels… and tell me about it…"*

Now, you notice that there is no suggestion, amongst all that urging, that the client should experience anything other than the feelings that have come up from the very depths of his own subconscious mind. There are some very powerful guiding and urging influences there, but no leads whatsoever. All we are doing is asking our client to have a closer look at something he has already told us about without being prompted. Of course, we are attaching importance to that event by the very fact that we are asking him to look at it in more detail, so we have to tread carefully. The urging part of it would not be undertaken until it was obvious that our client was indeed experiencing some sort of emotional recall.

Sometimes there would be a need to have a look at the situation again, to desensitise our client if it was a traumatic memory. Sometimes, though, it would be obvious from the client's demeanour that that simply was not necessary—he would mention it himself and comment on how it seemed totally unimportant now.

Not just in hypnosis

We need to be very careful at all times—and not just during the hypnosis part of each session—as far as leading and guiding are concerned. What we say to our client, and the way we say it, will have a profound effect upon his thought processes.

When we tell him how we work and what we plan to do, we need to make sure that he doesn't somehow gain the idea that we are looking for any particular type of event or circumstance. He will quite often be predisposed to believe that we will be seeking some sort of sexual situation. We should assure him that we have *absolutely no idea whatsoever*, at this stage, as to what might have caused his problems, only that we *know* that it's a bit of 'unfinished business' in the subconscious and that we know exactly how to find out exactly what that unfinished business actually is.

Any case history we use as an illustration of how we work, or to boost client confidence, should be as far removed from his particular set of symptoms as we can manage.

When we tell him about repression, we need to be careful not to indicate that it is likely to be of any specific nature.

Common sense

Once you've grasped the concept of guiding and not leading, and that the client will usually seek to relate everything you say to his own life and self, then the entire business of the language you use in therapy becomes a matter of an acquired common sense. It becomes easy!

Here is a somewhat humorous—and true—example of how directive language can be. There was a therapist, an ex-legal mind, who insisted that his clients always answered questions with a 'yes' or a 'no', seeking to keep therapy somewhat 'cut and dried'. All went well until a client stated emphatically that this was not always possible. A friendly but slightly heated discussion followed, with the therapist insisting that all questions could be brought down to an affirmative or negative answer, and that any other response was a form of resistance.

The client thought for a moment, then said: "All right, answer me this: Have you stopped beating your wife yet?"

Chapter 11

Understanding What the Client Doesn't Tell You

Much of the information in this chapter is mainly of use to the analytical or regression therapist, rather than to those who use suggestion or silence. But the 'rules' outlined here can be applied to a very large extent in any exchange with a client.

The way an individual behaves during a session will often provide huge clues as to the direction and/or source of her conflict. One of the major indicators comes from the way she tells you any form of personal history, be it in hypnosis or in a waking state—in the form of a lie. Memory tends to be dynamic—each recall of a specific event is slightly different if it is an honest recall, different aspects becoming apparent each time. If it is identical, or nearly identical, every time, it is *probably* a lie, though this may well be unintentional; it is likely that the client is simply telling you either what she told you during the last session, or the story that she has told so many times that she believes it to be fact. It is even possible that she has completely forgotten the *true* course of events.

It is easy to understand this when you recognise that if a story is fabricated or partly fabricated, there is only one thing to be recalled the next time—what was said last time. But if an event is being genuinely recalled in its entirety, and the event itself is being re-examined, then there are an awful lot more things to be remembered. What actually comes to mind is going to be affected by our mood at the time, by what has been discussed prior to the recall, what is going on in our lives at the time... and who we are telling the story to, of course.

Even the first time you hear a story, you can be aware of the fabrication; a true recall is interrupted with a few 'ums' and 'ers' and the odd "no, just a minute", "Oh, I should've said..." and so on. There will also be asides, interruptions and grammatical shifts: "The next-door neighbours used to invite me round—we found out later that her husband was an alcoholic—to play with their son." A 'fake' story is inclined to be more direct, less detailed, and more to the point, *because it is being told for a reason.* When you become aware that your client is telling you less than the truth, *you can be certain that she is talking about the source of at least part of her neurosis.*

The blatant lie

The out-and-out lie is told when there is an area of the psyche into which the client has no intention of allowing us to go—and a no-go area is, of course, **death** to any analytical process. These areas are usually associated with shame, perceived guilt, or intolerable embarrassment (either at the time of the event or at the recall of it), and will often be associated with 'private' bodily functions and/or sexuality. The biggest clue to the blatant lie comes from the changes in body language (discussed later in this chapter), and the therapist should be very aware that *it is a rehearsed evasion technique.* It will, in all probability, have been rehearsed and retold many times since the occurrence of the event with which it is associated (because of the urge to discharge the negative emotion), to allow your client to maintain integrity in some way. It is also highly possible that it is allowing your client to maintain her illness, since it is indicative of unfinished business.

It is with the RO personality (see Chapter Three) that this is most likely to show itself. The IA types are usually open and honest during therapy, and will willingly go back to a previous recall and search through it all again, looking for any missed details. The CE seldom bothers to lie at all, except to exaggerate, and then it is almost always obvious.

Body language

A major clue the client will unwittingly give us to an untruth is with body language. If what she is telling you is associated with some discomfort, there will often be a whole array of physical indicators. It is most noticeable with the CE personality, least (often barely discernible) with the RO. Some useful hints are as follows:

(1) The commonest indicator involves movements of the legs and feet; when the feet 'waggle', it is likely that the client *knows* that

there is a problem here but is currently unwilling or unable to confront it and wishes to run away, hence the movement.

(2) Jerks or twitches of the legs; similar to (1) though the client may be only dimly aware—or maybe even totally unaware—that there is negativity attached to the recall. These movements may be attached to an undischarged motor urge to run and may be quite vigorous. They will often be excused as a 'nerve twitch', along with the statement: "Oh, that's nothing, I've always had that."

(3) The thumbs suddenly being enclosed by the fingers, so that the hand makes what looks like a fist. This is usually associated with wanting to hide, or at least not be seen; an interesting point about this is that in Eastern hand reading (a little like palmistry) the thumb is considered to represent the Ego.

(4) Whole body tic, where there is a sudden small, but unmistakable, flurry of movement. Here, the client feels uncomfortable but does not really know why. She may be trying to 'shake it off'. Again this can be quite vigorous and there may be an attempt to disguise it by scratching or rubbing the face, etc.

(5) Any sudden change of body language speed, especially if your client is normally immobile then makes several small movements of the hands and arms (fighting) or feet (running). The reverse is also true, where your client is normally inclined towards animation or fidgeting but suddenly becomes very still.

Dealing with it (1)

Whichever of the above you observe, your response should always be the same; keep her on that same thought/concept and keep on 'digging' until you are happy that she has let go of the emotional state that is attached to the recall. The thing to watch for particularly is the same physical movements being repeated each time a particular recall is made. Bear in mind, though, that there will be occasions when body language clues turn out to be nothing more than random movement.

Dealing with it (2)

The rest of this chapter is of more use where the analytical process is being employed than with other styles of therapy.

Where you suspect that an evasion technique is being employed and your client seems determined to continue doing so, you need make her aware that you know about it (though without being obvious and especially without being accusatory) and point out that it will stop therapy from being effective. It is important that you help her realise that unless she 'spills the beans', the very thing that has brought her to you will stop her from getting relief from her symptoms.

Try a persuasive method first. Tell her exactly what you want; you want her to recall the actual event and tell it to you as it unfolds in her mind, rather than remember what she told you last time or what she might have told other people for various reasons. Explain that you want her to do this so that she does not miss anything which might need 'sorting out' before she can get better. Ask her questions to interrupt her thought pattern as she tells you the story, or go back to a mid-point and ask her to tell you a different aspect of it, or even to tell it in a different way.

Where she 'survives' this technique, then you will have to employ a slightly more confrontational approach... but as 'invisibly' as you can. A fairly easy and effective way to do this is to tell her a metaphorical story about a past client—and be sure that the client in front of you can identify with the imaginary one—who tried to 'plea bargain'. This client promised she would tell you everything, but it was not long before you realised that it had become a case of: "Well, anything except *that*!" Of course, you explain, a **'that'**, or anything like it, is necessarily going to be playing a huge part in the presenting symptoms and that until it is released, the subconscious will simply prohibit the conscious mind from going even near anything remotely connected with it. "Which is why the symptom exists in the first place," you would add. "Good old subconscious using a sledgehammer to crack a nut. As usual." Be sure to give a successful conclusion to your metaphorical case; the client was finally brave enough to talk about what had been troubling her (it is not necessary to say what it was) and felt **much** better afterwards!

It is also worth pointing out that you always *know* when something is being held back, because there are so many give-away signs 'to a psychologist'—but, of course, you say, you never let it show... Leave your client wondering whether or not you know about *her* 'something'.

It is a bit of a make-or-break situation, this, because some clients will simply not come back for their next session. On the other hand, if that does turn out to be the case, they probably would not have completed this type of therapy successfully anyway.

Types of recall

During the analytical session, a useful clue that something is 'near the surface' is when certain types of recall are evident. Two or more recalls of any of these types in the same session should be considered relevant:

(1) **Recall:** The 'cold' memory pattern—snowball fights, building snow men, being out in the snow, buying ice-cream, swimming, studying ice crystals, looking at icicles, ice-skating, swimming —anything to do with *cold*. Children feel cold when frightened. The reported recall may well have nothing to do with the trauma that is being avoided, but will often 'switch' dramatically and suddenly into an area of emotional distress. This will often be preceded by an ambiguous statement: "Dad's building me this snowman... I don't think I liked him very much."

   Action: Feeding back is very useful here. "And when Dad was building this snowman and you didn't like him very much... what else is there about that?" You can also take any of the statements and feed them back *in the same format in which they were spoken*, and add: "Now tell me more about that," or "And what happened then?"

(2) **Recall:** The good memory syndrome—a whole series of memories concerning happy times, times that were fun, times

of success, etc. Again, the reported recall may have little to do with the approaching recall of trauma. These memories can later be used as anchors to positive resources.

Action: Silence and waiting, or: "And when you had enjoyed all that fun… what happened then?" are probably the best responses here.

(3) **Recall:** The 'best friend' memory—repeated recalls of things done with a best friend, especially if the client was in a subservient role. Here, the reported recall almost certainly *does* have a bearing on the problem in the psyche.

Action: Waiting while your client is 'on' it. Otherwise, something like "And I wonder how (best friend's name) felt about that…" or "And when you were not with (best friend's name) what happened then?" Maybe even (though this is rather blatant): "And were you (best friend's name) best friend?" This often jogs a memory of feeling unloved or something similar.

(4) **Recall:** The 'perfect parent'—almost self-explanatory, this is where a parent is being reported as the best that ever lived, just before the realisation that there was a time when this individual's halo definitely 'slipped'!

Action: Just keep the client focused on that parent, *but do not be tempted to lead!*

(5) **Recall:** Lonely memories or 'nobody else is there' recalls.

Action: You can use these for session 'guides' if you need them. They are often 'next door' to areas of conflict. Come back to them if your client falls silent or cannot think of anything.

(6) **Recall:** Continual rainy-day memories tends to hint at trauma around the age of those memories. A similar thing is the memory of dark rooms, grey clothes, gloomy buildings, etc.

Action: Silence and waiting. Make a note of the reported age and if your client lapses into silence or a blank mind, then ask her to imagine being that age, then: "Tell me how it seems to be (age) years old."

Finally, a very informative circumstance that you can sometimes observe even before your client enters your office: she has brought along a friend or some other individual as moral support. This client will definitely be more difficult to get through a successful therapy, because she is seeking to avoid the responsibility of dealing with her problem on her own. She will be waiting for you to do the work and it is necessary to clarify at the outset that you have no special powers—you simply know how to *help her* find what she needs for herself. And even if you are using purely suggestion work, this holds true, for if she does not seek to operate upon your suggestions, no change will take place.

Chapter 12

Cinema—a Useful Dissociation Routine

This is an adaptation of a routine which has been in use by therapists for a good many years. Its main use is with the individual who is either frightened of what he might find during analysis/regression, or who has some trauma he needs to work through but simply cannot bear to look at.

Use an induction appropriate for the client and then proceed as follows:

Relax and go deeper now... and, as you do, imagine yourself sitting in a cinema... just you, no one else is there and you feel safe and comfortable... you are sitting in the most luxurious chair... notice where you are sitting in this place... maybe at the front or in the middle or to one side.

And imagine a huge screen right there, right in front of you... it's blank at the moment and has a sort of silvery shimmer, but soon, very soon, you will see something on that screen which is to your benefit... you may not understand the meaning of it at first but you needn't let that bother you... notice how soft and soothing the lighting is... it's an unusual and yet a very natural colour.

Now imagine actually stepping out of your body and standing in the aisle... just imagine standing in the aisle watching yourself sitting watching the blank screen and waiting... noticing how relaxed and comfortable you are... now imagine actually stepping out of that body standing in the aisle and find yourself standing at the back of the cinema watching yourself standing in the aisle, watching yourself sitting watching the blank screen... imagine stepping out of that body at the back of the cinema and going through some swing doors which are behind you.

Here you can see a brightly lit stairway leading up to the control room. Very slowly and very safely now make your way up the stairs and enter the control room... no one else may enter this place—just you and the sound of my voice... so make sure you close the door behind you... in front of you, see an opening in the wall, walk over to that opening and look down into the auditorium... see yourself standing at the back of the cinema watching yourself standing in the aisle, watching yourself sitting waiting... look back into the control room and see right there the projector with the spool of film in place... on the side of the projector are the control buttons similar to those which you might use on a video machine... you can see STOP, START, REWIND, FAST FORWARD and PAUSE... tell me, are the controls push-button or are they switches?

Wait for response.

What colour is the STOP button/switch?

Use client's description and wait for a response.

And is the START button/switch next to the STOP button/switch? Or is it above it, or below it, etc?

Get the location and ask the client to confirm it is there.

Now push the START button. You will hear the sound of the spools as they begin to go round and watch as the film begins to filter through on to the screen... go to the opening in the wall and tell me what you are seeing on the screen...

Using the dissociation technique

Be prepared for things like:

Client: *I can't find the START button.*

You will have noticed in the above script that detail is given about the location of the START button in order to pre-empt resistance here.

Client: *There's nothing on the screen.*

Use your imagination here and remember anything is possible, so suggest something like:

Therapist: Imagine the screen is a curtain like a roller-blind and as I count from five down to zero the curtain will rise and …

You may also hear:

Client: *The tape's broken.*

Therapist: *You have everything you need to fix it in the drawer on your left. Open it and take out the sticky tape, join the two ends together, that's right, see how easy it is.*

And so on …

Client: *The tape's jammed.*

Therapist: *Is it jammed in the machine or on the spool?*

Get detail and fix it with your client. Remember that whatever your client needs to carry out the repair you will make available in the control room.

Client: *It's all fuzzy.*

Therapist: *Use the controls and bring it into focus, etc.*

It is impossible to cover every eventuality, so let your own ingenuity run wild where necessary!

Chapter 13

The Telephone Technique for the 'Non-visual' Client

This technique has many uses but it is more suited to the auditory and kinaesthetic-modality types. It can be used for anyone who really finds it difficult to get in touch with the unconscious mind. It is so simple that, in some ways, perhaps the reason that it works so effectively is that it requires little planning on the part of the therapist.

One of the key things to bear in mind when using this method of extracting information from the unconscious mind is that it is necessary for you to give no previous knowledge of what is about to happen. Also, it is done very quickly because that avoids the client's rationalisation of what is about to happen. The most useful purpose it serves is either to extract new information, or to confirm something which the client has difficulty in believing. It can also be added to the ideo-motor method of confirmation as a back up.

A non-visual induction will work best here, perhaps just dealing with the body and the individual organs of the body, and including a progressive relaxation if the client is fairly tense. You could even actually ask the client to take that tension still further before she lets it all go and really becomes more focused on physical relaxation.

Having completed the induction, the use of a physical-style deepener is a good idea; if you choose to use a visual deepener for any reason, though, be sure that it is very simple—keeping the client more and more aware of her own body. The routine works best when trance is induced at a fairly fast rate because the auditory personality group—as well as those who have very little visualisation ability—needs to be mentally occupied; you will need to use a script in which you are delivering a vast number of words even though there may be several repetitions of phrases.

So having done an induction which is appropriate to your client, begin by just highlighting the nature of the client's particular problem—the one thing which perhaps you have struggled to extract from her. The two examples given below are fairly simple but enormously successful.

Case study 1

We are going to look at an example of a client who was suffering with constant headaches. This condition was actually disturbing the therapy itself and so it was something which had to be removed before proper progress could be made.

The client was a young professional male in a very pressurised and responsible position in a family business, where it involved a lot of work with figures and marketing services. He was single and had recently moved from his parents' house and set up his own home. The headaches started not long after this move.

During free-association in therapy there seemed to be great difficulty in actually overcoming the barrier of the headache and it was decided to deal with this problem independently:

> *Therapist: (Name), as you relax there, wondering about headache and how it is affecting your work, we could do something quite useful for you. Is that okay?*
>
> *Client: Yes.*
>
> *Therapist: I'd like you to imagine a telephone, one of those old ones that has no dial. Perhaps you may have seen one—or can remember now—the type of telephone which has no dial.*
>
> *Client: Yes.*
>
> *Therapist: And when you look at the telephone which has no dial, I'd like you to tell me what colour that telephone is because it may be any colour that you choose. It could be light or dark.*
>
> *Client: It's a black one, like the old-fashioned type.*
>
> *Therapist: Good. That's right. Just for a moment and before we continue, think once more—and perhaps you know what purpose*

headache serves—so that you can end headache without the need to continue to find the cause.

Client: *No. I have no idea why my headaches are there.*

Therapist: *That's fine. So now we can go ahead and find out what purpose headache is serving. So that once we have found out we can then work to eliminate headache. In a moment I shall ask you to pick up that telephone and I will ask you a question which I would like you to repeat in your mind and to speak into that telephone. Then I want you to tell me, word for word, exactly what you hear in the earpiece of the telephone, because, you see, (name), the telephone is now connected to your unconscious mind and it is probably the most direct way of discovering now the cause of headache. Be comfortable now as you go still deeper to discover that you are more relaxed. And slowly now pick up the telephone, holding it towards your left ear. Good. That's right. And I'd like you to repeat the question into the mouth-piece, though you only need do this in your mind. This is the question I want you to ask: UNCONSCIOUS, WHAT NEEDS TO HAPPEN FOR MY HEADACHES TO CEASE?*

At this time there was about a 30-second to 40-second delay. And then the answer was amazing because of its simplicity.

Client: *Be true to yourself.*

Therapist: *And, unconscious, how is it that (name) is not true to himself?*

Client: *He is working in a place where he should not be working. In a place that's causing frustration.*

Therapist: *Fine. Thank you for letting us know this. Unconscious, in order for (name) and I to work better together I would need for the headaches to be reduced sufficiently in order that (name) can allow the information contained deep within you to be made available to him. Is that agreeable?*

After quite a pause the answer came up:

Client: *Yes.*

> **Therapist:** *Now I'd like a confirmation so that (name) too under-stands now that this will happen by arranging that the pointing finger—the YES finger—of his right hand, the YES finger, rises sufficiently and involuntarily.* (Of course, the ideo-motor response has been prepared prior to the session)

The index finger then rose up. The client, quite surprised by all this, began to talk about his discontent about working with his father. The therapy then continued more freely and he was able to recall situations and talk about his father's total inability to show him any affection and any praise whatsoever even though this young adult was running a multi-million-pound business.

Case study 2

This client had suffered with a combination of frustration, sexual promiscuity and then, at the other extreme, sexual dysfunction. During her therapy she discovered that the genital itching and soreness—from which she continually suffered—constantly kept taking her to a scene where she was abused by a member of her family. Now this was someone to whom she was very close but who had died by the time she was about nine years old. The abuse took place at the age of approximately five or six years old.

At the end of the therapy, the client was really determined that these events did not take place and asked us for our opinion. As is usual, she was told that we do not give opinions because that is not what we are here for; but several different links and connections that she had already made were pointed out to her. For instance, that the headaches which she was getting were linked to her father shouting at her. That the kleptomania from which she was suffering was linked to her getting attention by stealing money... and yet she still did not want to acknowledge the one thing which led to the discomfort in her genital area.

Now, interestingly enough, there were a few other key indicators. For example, when she was away from therapy and spoke to the widowed spouse of the abuser, saying politely how nice it would be if he were back now, she actually felt discomfort about what she had spoken about during one of the sessions.

Again, you should not pass comment—the only words which you can say are something like *"ah ha"* or virtually repeat what the client has said. In this case a very rapid response was made:

> **Therapist:** *Do you really want to know what happened? There is a way of knowing right now.*

The client replied that she did and was soon being asked to imagine the telephone with no dial, as in the previous case. Then:

> **Therapist:** *On the other end of that telephone you will hear a child's voice and I want you to ask the question word for word. Tell me when you have that telephone.*

> **Therapist:** *What colour is that telephone?*

> **Client:** *Red.*

> **Therapist:** *Pick up the telephone now, holding it to your left ear and ask the following question, just in your thoughts, in your mind only. I'd like to know whether little (name) is there on the other end of that telephone?*

> **Client:** *Yes.*

> **Therapist:** *I'd like to know from little (name) whether what she has shown adult (name), really happened?*

> **Client:** *Yes.*

> **Therapist:** *I'd like to know from little (name) whether she knows why adult (name) isn't believing her?*

> **Client:** *It's too painful and she still loves Uncle Tom.*

> **Therapist:** *I'd like to know from little (name) whether you can find a way of keeping the love and letting go of the pain?*

> **Client:** *I don't know.*

> **Therapist:** *That's fine. I'd like to know if there's another way you can show adult (name) what happened by giving adult (name) even more information?*
>
> **Client:** *Yes.*
>
> **Therapist:** *That's good.*

Over the course of the next few sessions more and more information became available to the client, and when this seemed complete, the therapy was completed thus:

> **Therapist:** *I need for you to know something that your unconscious mind has been trying to tell you for a long time. You need to have an understanding about what happens to us as children, to understand the effects which only you can either accept or reject. But it is this acceptance of your true self which will liberate you.*

An alternative

Another way of using this very direct method is to bypass the conscious mind and the unconscious mind, and take away the responsibility from the client for a while. The technique is slightly different here because it requires more imagination; the picture which you will need to create in the client's mind is that of a telephone exchange similar to the ones used in the forties and fifties although, of course, you could use a more up-to-date one. The exchange represents the workings of the inner mind and we are going interrupt the communication which has been going on between unconscious and conscious.

Be as free as you can in describing the exchange and in allowing the client to imagine a system which has plugs and cables (the dolls-eye switchboard). Show the client that there is communication going from one side of the switchboard to the other, and in every area where there is incongruence present there will be a light to show this. This will indicate that there is a communication going from one part of the unconscious mind to one part of the conscious mind—and show the client that she can interrupt this communication and listen in to what the unconscious mind is trying to tell the conscious mind. The technique can be adapted in many different ways and once it has been used five or six times you will be able to find the right way to create the right image.

The entire routine can also work extremely well if the telephone is replaced by a computer, a good method to use with younger clients who may never have seen the older style of telephones or exchange.

Chapter 14

The Fibre-optics Technique to Deal with Discomfort

This technique will ideally suit clients in whom the symptom manifests itself in a physical way and where the client is experiencing discomfort which has no medical explanation. It is equally useful with non-physical symptoms which disturb the client, as well as with clients who experience difficulty with verbal communication.

It is important that if a client has only recently experienced the pain or discomfort he should first be asked if he has consulted a doctor and, if not, should be advised to do so.

Fibre-optics script

Use an appropriate induction and then proceed as follows:

"It is interesting when you realise how, over the last few years, so many discoveries and so many advances have been made and are possible. And how so many have been made to make your life so much easier—making it possible to improve your everyday life in ways which are almost unimaginable.

*"I was thinking about that great new discovery called fibre optics—a branch of optics dealing with the transmission of light and other important information through fibres or thin rods of glass or some other transparent material of high refractive index. I am sure you will remember the past and will recall that wire was used to send information from one place to another, like on a telephone, when you can talk while sitting and relaxing. And even before that, people would send messages with smoke signals to tell each other about important things and perhaps that's where that saying comes from about: **There is no smoke without fire**.*

"I don't know … but perhaps you do.

"If light or other information is admitted in a kind of code at one end of a fibre, it can and will travel through the fibre with very low loss, even if the fibre is curved and that might not be logical. The scientific principle on which this transmission of light depends is that of total internal reflection. The fibre is so fine that you could get hundreds of them through the eye of a needle. That's amazing. That's right.

"In order to avoid losses through the scattering of light by impurities on the surface of the fibre, the optical-fibre core is covered with a glass layer of much lower refractive index. This makes resistance a thing of the past so that the end-reflections will occur effortlessly at the interface of the glass-fibre and the cladding... also, bundles of several thousands of very thin fibres, assembled precisely side by side and optically polished at their ends, can be used to transmit images and other important information. Each point of the image projected on one face of the bundle is reproduced at the other end of the bundle, reconstituting the image, which you can observe through a magnifier. Image-transmission by optical fibres is widely used in medical instruments for viewing inside the human body—which, coincidentally, is how we think they discovered that cells talk to each other. Optical fibres are used for laser surgery, in facsimile systems, in computer graphics and in many other applications and, perhaps, even on a television screen.

"And as you think about the benefits of optical fibre you could wonder what next will be possible...

"Now I'd like you to place your awareness on that part of your body which has been causing you that discomfort, that painful feeling, that unwanted feeling which you described to me."

Use all the details from your client's information ensuring that, where possible, the language used is as near as possible to the client's description and begin to slow the pace down at this point.

"You could imagine or pretend—and it doesn't matter which—an invisible fibre, just like an optical fibre. And take one end and place it on just the right place and I'm sure you will remember where that place is. And place the other end in the screen of your mind, that's right, the same screen that's used by your imagination.

"And as you do, you will, because you choose to, allow that part of your body to show that part of your mind which needs the information, just what it's doing there… and, more importantly, what purpose it needed to serve and why—so as to then let that feeling go… just allow that experience now to come uppermost in your mind on the screen in your imaginative mind and as soon as you experience it through any of your powerful imaginative circuits… your sight… or sound… or feelings… or taste… or smell… or sense…

"And it doesn't matter which or all come to you first—just tell me anything and everything which is being transmitted to you… when you next hear the number 'three'… one, two, three."

Method

The example given below (an actual case) assumes that no medical solution has been found and that the client has had a painful symptom for some time without explanation. Take time, using clean language, to isolate the problem area and its effects. For example:

Therapist: The pain in your chest which you described—is it within the area of your ribs?

Client: Yes.

Therapist: Can you be more specific?

Client: It's by my heart.

Therapist: And what does it do for you?

Client: It hurts like something is going to break.

Therapist: Shall we find out what it's doing there?

The therapy commenced at this point and took the client to a scene at a bar where he met his girlfriend. The client thought that he was about eighteen or nineteen years old. Then:

Therapist: *What are you doing there?*

Client: *It's that day.*

Therapist: *What day?*

Client: *It's the day she told me.*

Therapist: *The day that she has told you what?*

Client: *That she doesn't want to see me any more. She says her Mum thinks that it's better that she goes to university. But I love her. She's broken my heart.*

The therapy, working through the situation, continued until the screen (in the mind) was clear of any negative feelings. The example shown here is quite simple but very significant in that the client's unconscious mind revealed several clues in the spoken word.

Sometimes an element of resistance sets in if the therapist does not sound convincing with the script, so rehearse the script several times before using it.

On the subject of resistance, the following are some examples and techniques to overcome some of the most obvious forms of resistance.

Client	*Therapist*
The cable has broken.	*That's okay, don't let that bother you, there's plenty more. Let's start again, now.*
There is nothing there.	*What colour is nothing, etc?*
I can't make the connection.	*What stops you?*
I can't see the screen.	*That's right, it takes a few moments—like when you turn the television on.*
It's hazy.	*Find the control switch.*

It's nothing.	*I know but still tell me.*
It's horrible.	*Tell me about horrible.*
I don't want to see it.	*What is it that you don't want to see?*
No.	*What No?*

The list is endless but the end result is always the same—it only works.

Use any techniques you feel appropriate to overcome any barriers and to desensitise the client should the experience become too painful. Most importantly know and understand that the client's own processes are working with you to help him.

Chapter 15

The Cylinder Technique to Free your Client's Emotions

This is an invaluable routine to use with those clients who have either trouble in expressing emotion, or difficulty in feeling some or all emotional responses to begin with.

Use an appropriate induction and then proceed as follows:

"Now that you are relaxed, calm and peaceful, I would like you to focus on something for me. I would like you to listen very quietly to the sound of my voice because in a moment you are going to do something for yourself... something which is going to be very beneficial to you, something which you have wanted to do for a long time... something which will benefit you now and always... and your unconscious mind knows what it is that needs to be done and is already preparing to do this for you.

"So just relax in this warm and comfortable position and enjoy this lovely feeling of total and complete relaxation... just imagine a safe and warm darkness, a velvety darkness... and imagine, in this warm and welcoming darkness, a soft and gentle light... it could even be a coloured light—maybe green, or yellow, or blue. Your unconscious mind knows which colour it is and it will show you. Imagine as you begin to focus on the light that you see more lights in the distance... as if you are in a corridor, a corridor in the deepest part of your unconscious mind.

"As you focus down the corridor you begin to feel yourself walking down the corridor. Down this long and softly-lit corridor—perhaps it's carpeted with a soft, smooth, fluffy carpet... as you walk down deeper to the deepest part of your unconscious mind, imagine there, right there in the distance, a very special sort of door, a very strong door. It could be made of steel or perhaps it's made of wood. Your unconscious mind knows what it's made of. As you move closer and closer and go deeper and deeper towards the door, you can see and feel the door, what it's made of and how strong it is... and as you move

still closer to it you see something written on the door… it says: EMOTIONS CONTROL ROOM.

"In a moment you will be able to enter this room and you will be able to examine and see that everything is functioning and that every-thing is free-flowing… that all blockages have been removed, because your body needs to have free-flowing emotions. Like a river flowing through a valley… and as that river gently flows through that valley, so it feeds and nourishes the valley, and keeps everything healthy and fertile.

"You see, the water which flows provides for all life and it heals and repairs all the valley… just as nature intended… nature makes sure that the whole valley is kept healthy and alive… as the river spreads itself across the valley by having brooks and streams, it feeds the valley.

"Imagine, now, that you have entered the EMOTIONS CONTROL ROOM. Close the door behind you because no one else may enter—just you, and the sound of my voice. Inside the room there is a row of steel cylinders. Focus on the row of cylinders. See how strong they are, made of the most solid, stainless steel and notice how each one has an open top… notice also that each cylinder has writing on it. Soon you will be able to see what each cylinder has written on it.

"Each cylinder has a tap, or perhaps it's a valve, or it could be a sort of control mechanism. You will know which it has as you move closer to each one… and those taps or valves should all be flowing gently down into a large opening—a sort of gully… to succeed, we need to make sure that every emotion is free-flowing…

"There may have been times in the years gone by when emotions had to be turned off… but, you know, you should go through life with all the taps and valves turned on… because, if a pipe gets blocked or a mechanism gets stuck the cylinder will overflow and the contents will go everywhere, making the floor slippery and you will be unable to walk through life…so just look at the cylinders now. See each one and the emotion it contains and tell me which one is turned off… if all the cylinders are on and free-flowing… good! Otherwise, just go to the one that is off or stuck and free it."

Any resistance is likely to be minimal here. The following illustrates how to deal with it easily and effectively.

> **Client:** *I can't.*

> **Therapist:** *Find a way.*

You may suggest using a spanner or hammer or rock, etc. at this point to assist your client. When the freeing-off process is complete, proceed as follows:

> **Therapist:** *Would you like to know why the cylinder was turned off/blocked/stuck (etc.).* (Use your client's description here.)

Or:

> **Therapist:** *Tell me of a time when you held back that emotion. Focus on it. Let it rise to the surface. Feel it, etc...*

From here, it is a simple matter of helping your client work through whatever situation or circumstance she finds herself recalling. If she gets 'stuck' at any point, then you can take her back to the cylinder that was stuck and ask her if it is free-flowing yet.

Chapter 16

Two Easy Methods of Accessing Repressed Emotion

Boxes

The 'boxes' method can be astonishingly effective, especially if you have used the 'private place' routine (Chapter Six) in one of your early sessions and placed the boxes in there already. If you have not, then take your client down some steps in his mind at the end of a suitable induction, then proceed as follows:

"Focus and notice a door. This is the door to your private room where only you and the sound of my voice may enter. Imagine opening the door. It's a most wonderful feeling as you enter your private room— welcoming and safe. Close the door behind you, no-one else may enter… just you and the sound of my voice.

"Slowly look around your room—it feels so peaceful and relaxing… in your room focus and notice a chair, the most comfortable chair you have ever seen… a chair of your own choosing… your unconscious mind will show you the right image for you… maybe it's soft and feathery, with pillows and cushions in different colours and different fabrics… or perhaps it's firmer, with a floral pattern… just imagine how much more relaxed you can become and, as you do, relax and go deeper down into complete calmness… just imagining yourself lazily sinking into that chair.

"You feel safe in your room as you become more and more peaceful inside… listening lazily and comfortably to the sound of my voice. And as you listen to the sound of my voice so your comfort-level increases more and more… a bond growing and developing between you and the sound of my voice… so you can feel safe in your room with all your favourite things around you.

"And next to you on your right is a low table… and on that table are some boxes… take a little time to examine not only the table but also the assortment of boxes. All different colours, shapes and sizes. A mixture of boxes—all individual, all different…

> *"I'd like you to tell me: how many boxes can you see there?"*

Allow client time, and watch for REM (Rapid Eye Movement).

> *"Good… choose one. Just reach out and pick it up… what colour is it? Is it large or small? As you hold it, does it feel heavy or light? Does it feel like there is more than one object inside? Notice the way it opens, in a way which is characteristic of you… now open the box and take out whatever is inside.*
>
> *"Hold it in your left hand.*
>
> *"What is it that you are holding?*
>
> *"Look at X closely… focus all your attention on that X… hold it in your left hand and really feel it…"*

Brief pause.

> *"Now I want you to close both your hands around X… and imagine you are going to close your eyes still holding X… on the count of 'three', imagine opening your eyes in a different place and a different time…"*

If client opens eyes, reinforce eye-closure.

> *"One, two, three. Where do you find yourself?"*

Case fragments

Here are two fragments of case histories showing how this routine works. It is not important that the therapist's conscious mind should understand precisely why the client has made whatever connection he finds; the important thing is that that client accesses repressed emotional states.

Sally counted six boxes—the one she chose to pick up was a small, wooden box with a sort of flowery spiral carved into the lid. The box felt light and contained only one object, and the lid opened in a very simple way (her own words). From the box she took out a small, old, brass key.

On the count of 'three' she found herself at school at the age of six being bullied by another girl. She had a feeling in her tummy as if it were going round and round. This girl had continued to bully Sally for a very long time to the point where we found the child in bed crying because she was in fear of going to school. The only help she got from her mother was:

"It's very simple—stay out of her way."

Jake counted three boxes—he chose a brown cardboard box, the size of a shoe box, which felt quite heavy and contained more than one object. The lid just lifted off and he found a pair of roller-skates, when he started to cry. He said: "They're a birthday present from my Dad but he's never here."

Jake continued to cry till he was exhausted.

The object(s) in the box will usually be related in some way to the memory that is accessed as a result, though frequently this will not be so. The subconscious mind often works with symbols that are specific and personal to the individual, and one person's representation of a problem may be totally different from that of someone else.

Keys

This technique is very helpful for use with a 'stuck' client in analysis and/or where there is a guilt complex in operation. It is interactive and very difficult for your client to resist, since it relies on accessing subconscious thought processes for the entire session. It has the added advantage that, as soon as there is acceptance of, and subsequent interaction with, the fantasy of the situation, then the conscious critical faculty is automatically by-passed.

You can either have your client collect the bunch of keys from the 'private place' (Chapter Six), or have him relaxing in any place he likes to be: on the beach, in a park, strolling through a beautiful country estate or garden, ambling lazily along a country lane... anywhere that feels *good* to him. It can be daytime or night time, hot or cold (or warm), good weather or bad weather—whatever seems right to your client. Let him invent the scene. Have him find the bunch of keys lying around and observe that it is 'just a bunch of keys'... except for one, the special one which is very obviously the most important. *Do not, at this stage, give the client any idea what the keys are for or why you are doing this technique. We need a sense of mystery and wondering.*

Ask him to describe the keys; how many there are (you could limit them, but clients will seldom give you an unworkably high number and it will often be three or five), what they are like, how heavy they feel, etc., and how he can tell that the important one *is* the important one. Make sure that he has identified that one clearly enough in his mind that *you* can see it when he describes it.

Wherever he is when he comes into possession of the keys, have him continue on his way (or go outside first if he is in the private place) until he finds a building that he just *knows* the keys are for. This should happen fairly quickly; if it does not, encourage him to look around him. You can even ask why he cannot see it. Do not accept "don't know". If he is not looking in the right place, tell him to look in the right place now.

Talk him inside and get a description of where he is—the type of room, corridor, hall, etc.—and say that those keys will eventually let him find the most important place in this building, the place where there is the reason for his problem. That place can only be unlocked by the most important key of all, and might be a cellar or an attic or just an ordinary room; it might be at the top or bottom of some stairs, at the end of a corridor or hall, or just on the other side of a door from any other room. Wherever he finds it, that door is the door to the secret place in his mind, the place where the answer is, and he can only go in there when he has explored the other places that his keys will let him go.

Now take him through the building, unlocking doors as he goes and leaving the key in the lock each time. Each room contains something that is important to him; a picture, a thought, a sound, an item, a written note, etc. Explore each thoroughly, using free association if necessary. You are likely to find emotional releases from time to time, sometimes even full abreaction, since he will be continually accessing thought processes and memory traces associated with the cause of his symptoms.

The last key and the last room needs careful handling; when he finds it, have him turn the key in the lock, then pause in quietness for a few seconds (to allow anticipation to rise). Then ask him if he is ready to enter the room—it is important to get his agreement. Tell him he must tell you immediately what he finds there and when you judge it to be the right moment urge him with: "It's time! Go in there now! Do it! Go on! Tell me—tell me what's there!"

This almost always produces, at the very least, a strong link to the neurosis, at best a headlong rush into the heart of it!

There are a few possibilities that can be generated by resistance. Ways of dealing with these are:

Client: No keys fit this door.

Therapist: Maybe it's the important one—come back to it later on.

Client: I can't see any other door from this room.

Therapist: Go back out of the room by the door you came in. (Repeat this if necessary—if he ends up outside the building, have him search around the outside for another door.)

Client: It's too dark to see.

Therapist: Move your hand along the wall until you find a light switch.

Client: This room's completely empty.

Therapist: Look at the walls. What do you see there? What colour are they? What does that colour mean to you?

Client: This corridor is too long—I can't see the end of it.

Therapist: Just keep on walking… the longer the corridor, the closer you are getting to the secret.

Client: There's a big hole in the floor.

Therapist: Jump into it—tell me where you find yourself.

Client: I'm back outside.

Therapist: Walk around the walls until you find another door. Or perhaps you can see an outbuilding... Tell me what you see.

Client: Only the most important key fits this room. (before the other rooms have been explored).

Therapist: Then remember where that room is and come back to it later. Remember something about the room and tell me about it. (This is so that you can take him back there later.)

Resistance on finding the 'secret' room may appear:

Client: I can't turn the key.

Therapist: I'll help you. There—it's turning now! Can you feel that?

Client: There's nothing there.

Therapist: All right—just give me your first impression to the things I ask you. (Now continue as shown in Chapter Nine).

Client: I'm stuck—I can't go in.

Therapist: Because...? (Do not accept 'Don't know'.)

Client: There's somebody in there—I'm frightened.

Therapist: Tell me who's there / And you're frightened because...?

There are other resistive statements that may be made, but those listed are the most likely. The important thing is for you to find a way to actually *use* the resistance in your client's favour in some way, rather than to allow the resistance to dominate the proceedings.

Handled properly, this routine will build up an air of mystery, anticipation and expectation from the beginning. Your client is no longer searching through consciousness for that elusive memory, and as a result logical intervention is far less likely than with some other uncovering techniques.

Chapter 17

*The Slide Show—A Powerful Device for Recall
or Dissociation*

The technique described in this chapter is a powerful aid to recall for clients in analytical therapy whose memories are sparse, or where they seem unable to free-associate. It also provides an exceptionally effective dissociation technique to help those individuals who need to 'work through' a trauma but who find it too distressing to approach by even triple-dissociative methods. An inventive therapist will no doubt find other ways in which it can be used, for it will lend itself well to the 'swish' technique, as well as therapy for motivation, goal-setting, social phobias, and other behavioural situations.

The main reason it works so well is simply that it is an anchor to the visualisation process.

'Setting up' routine

Whatever the reason for its employment, the introduction to the client will be the same, preferably delivered during hypnosis:

> *"Right, (name), I'd like you to imagine one of those slide projectors that people used to show their holiday snaps on before everybody had video…and I'd like you to imagine, as well, that it has one of those remote control buttons connected to the machine by a cable, and you have the control button in your hand…"*

So now your client already has the sense that she is in control of the situation, essential if you are seeking to approach an area of trauma. From here on, we handle each situation differently.

Dissociation

Used carefully, this can produce complete desensitisation to a traumatic incident, usually in one or two sessions—though in severe cases you may need more to bring it to completion. It is also possible that you will need to repeat the process a couple of times or so for some clients.

> *"And you probably remember those cartridges that held all the slides... well, I want you to imagine that you're holding just such a cartridge. The cartridge contains slides of that situation that has disturbed you so much over the years, right up to the moment when it was finally over and you were safe again... but it's okay, because they're nowhere near the projector yet and you have hold of them. So that situation is totally under your control. In your mind, now, turn it over and over; let yourself feel that cartridge and those slides, feeling just how thin each one is... noticing how easy it would be for them to just fall out..."*

There is an enormous amount going on here! Having hold of the situation, being safe, control, turning it over in your mind, feeling it, each slide being thin (small), and how easy it would be to let it go (fall out). Continue:

> *"How does that feel?"*

Wait for "Okay" and do more, if necessary, until you get it. Then:

> *"Good...right, we'll just pop that cartridge into the projector, but it's still okay, because you have the control button and you're totally in control... Now, this is a special projector, in that it has a colour control, and a volume control... and both are turned right down, so those slides will be in black and white only, with no sound. Would you like to see them from the beginning, or would you like to go backwards through them?"*

You appear to be giving your client choice and control here. You are *not* offering the option to not see the slides, but it will feel to your client that she has agreed to look at them. Some clients will want to 'watch the show' in reverse order, first of all seeing the time when they were safe again. Others will want to start at the beginning. Whichever she indicates ask her to press the slide projector control button, then ask her to tell you what she can see. In a very severe case, you could ask her to let you know when she is ready to press the button to see the first slide. Work through each scene as much as is needed for your client to 'push the button' to change the slide, until you get to the 'biggie'—that's where you have to eventually aim at keeping her there until she can view it comfortably, although you can let her move on to the next one fairly quickly, at first.

From now on, it is plain—and obvious—sailing! When she can go through the whole event forwards, do it again increasing the colour, resolution, sound, and finally, convert each 'slide' into a seamlessly joined video/film that she can 'float into' when she feels ready to do so. This last step is probably the most difficult for her and it definitely helps if you let her take that control button with her!

Analytical recall

Here we are going to use this technique to 'trigger' free association. There are many times when a client either claims to be able to remember nothing, or when she brings logic to bear upon each memory, or presents chronological memories only. With this technique, you can arrest that process by the simple expedient of asking your client to push the button to see what the next slide is. As with many of our methods, it relies heavily for its success on the imagery with which we present it to our client. Start with the 'setting up' routine, then continue:

> *"Now, I want you to pretend that this slide projector is already loaded with a cartridge absolutely stuffed full of all sorts of scenes from your early years… but there **is** a tiny snag…somebody's gone and got the slides all mixed up, so we can have absolutely no idea in which order they will appear. You'll probably see yourself at, oh, I don't know… say, seven years old in one of them, then the next might be from twelve, or four, or thirteen, or perhaps as young as only two years old…maybe you'll see yourself at school, or with your friends one moment, and the next one will be on holiday with Mum and Dad… who knows. We shall see…"*

Be very careful not to stress any of the ages or places you mention, since it may easily be taken as an indicator of where you believe the problem to be. This paragraph is a wonderful excuse for you to feed back any information you already have concerning your client's formative years. Continue:

> *"Now before you push that control button for the first slide... this is a very special slide projector, because just as soon as that picture appears on the screen in front of you... it becomes a moving, living, brightly coloured thing with sounds and smells, and feelings and even tastes...it becomes almost like real life, because, of course, what you're going to be looking at **was** real life, back then, back there, when you were just a child..."*

This is more scene-setting and will deepen the hypnotic state quite well. It also tells your client that you want to keep to memories, rather than imagination, as well as making it difficult for her to merely tell you a *translation* of her recall rather than the recall itself.

This is the: *"I remember school sports day..."* instead of: *"I remember coming last in the high jump, on school sports day"* syndrome. As an alternative to overcome this, try using imaginary video film that keeps on stopping, instead of a slide projector, impressing on the client that she has to tell you about the single frame of film she has seen, rather than what the event turned out to be.

Having fired your client's imagination, you continue by asking her to press the button for the first time and to tell you straight away what she finds herself looking at.

Now you—and your client—are on your way!

Behavioural change

There are several ways of tackling this, one of which is via an adapted version of the swish technique (the 'Moment-of-anxiety' picture automatically triggering the projector to move on to the 'Moment-of-achievement' picture, then the client pushing the button to go to the 'Neutral-place' picture, repeated several times with different scenes each time). A useful alternative, though, is to have the slides arranged in order from now to when the desired behaviour change has been achieved, having your client focusing on the steps in between the two. As with the dissociative technique, some clients may prefer to view the process in reverse; whichever they choose, be certain that they have fully grasped what their subconscious mind is offering them at each step of the way.

Part Three

Non-analytical Work

Chapter 18

A Day in a Life—an Aid to Focusing

This is a very useful idea to have to hand when your client experiences difficulty in speaking about himself. In fact, what happens with this technique is that you become the client and your client is asked to speak to you about yourself. By reading through the following example you will gain a clearer understanding of the way in which this technique can be used.

A woman has arrived for therapy not knowing what her problem is but she feels that something is definitely not right in her life just now.

> **Therapist:** *What I would like you to do, (name), is to pretend that I am you and that you are going to tell me about a typical day in my life. About what time do I get up?*

> **Client:** *Maybe eight or eight-thirty, somewhere about that time.*

> **Therapist:** *Okay and what do I do first? Do I make a drink or go to the loo or have a shower?*

> **Client:** *You can't be bothered to shower, you just go to the kitchen and make a drink and while the kettle boils, you feed the cat, Loopy, he's lovely.*

> **Therapist:** *Then what do I do?*

> **Client:** *Have a coffee and a few cigarettes.*

> **Therapist:** *And what am I thinking about while I have a coffee and a few cigarettes?*

> **Client:** *Nothing, really.*

> **Therapist:** *What am I feeling?*

Client: Same. Nothing, sort of frozen, I guess.

Therapist: Then what do I do next?

Client: Well, you have a bit of a wash and get dressed for work.

Therapist: Do I like my job?

Client: You don't like it much.

Therapist: What don't I like about it?

Client: It's boring.

Therapist: What time do I leave the house to go to work?

Client: Nine-o-clock.

Therapist: How do I get there?

Client: Walk. It's only down the road.

Therapist: What's the first thing I do when I get to work?

Client: Sort out the post. Then you do the photocopying and take it round.

Therapist: Do I speak to anyone?

Client: Only if there's a mistake.

Therapist: Do I have a coffee-break?

Client: Whenever you want. Sometimes you eat your lunch before lunch-time.

Therapist: Do I share my office with anyone?

Client: You're not in an office, you're in the post room downstairs on your own.

Therapist: *How do I feel about that?*

Client: *Okay. Well, a bit bored sometimes, so you have the radio on.*

Therapist: *What time do I go home?*

Client: *Five-o-clock.*

Therapist: *Do I walk home?*

Client: *Yes.*

Therapist: *Is anyone there when I get home?*

Client: *No, but Loopy always comes to meet you.*

Therapist: *What's the first thing I do when I get home?*

Client: *Put the telly on.*

Therapist: *What do I think about my life, (name)?*

Client: *Lonely and boring.*

The client has just told you exactly what he needs to resolve. You could begin now to use free association with the themes of *'a lonely time'* or *'a boring time'*.

Chapter 19

Table-Top Therapy™*

*Georges Philips & Lyn Buncher 1994

This technique is designed for clients who are primarily left-brain motivated, who are rational, logical and who feel the need to be in control. It works particularly well for those who are finding themselves behaving in a way that is unpalatable to them, but which they seem powerless to control. It also finds a great use in dealing with relationship difficulties.

At all times your position as a therapist should be to take an unbiased stand even though it may appear from the outset that there is a particularly destructive side at the table.

With this technique, the most destructive side (that is to say, the most resistant side) must be given the opportunity to express her feelings totally and to show her reasons for her behaviour. It is not unlikely that there will be an age difference in this manifestation of that part of the personality—the younger the image, the more powerful the influence.

Occasionally more than two images will appear, in which case improvise by simply stating that the appropriate number of chairs will be there at the table. Although it is possible that the client will create a very vivid room and table, the fewer the distractions, however, the more focused the client will become.

Table-top script

Use a standard relaxation induction and then proceed as follows:

"Imagine a dark room. Imagine a lamp hanging over a table and, as you focus, notice that there are at least 3 chairs round the table. Now I would like you to imagine yourself sitting in the central chair. Take your time and make yourself comfortable. That's right.

"First I would like you to take some time to listen to the sound of my voice. And, in particular, in your own way, listen to the things which

I shall ask of you so that you can gain a greater understanding of the problems you are facing in your life. For a while I would like you to be just a witness... without any particular point of view or thought, without prejudging... just seeing and listening as you are now, like an overseer of events. That's right.

"Now look to your left and notice an image of yourself walking towards the table...this is the part which feels X symptom or emotion... just see this part come and sit on your left."

Wait for confirmation—preferably non-verbal.

"Now look to your right... and notice another part of yourself coming towards the table. This is the part which feels Y symptom or emotion."

Wait for confirmation—preferably non-verbal.

(There will always be two sets of emotions or symptoms, at least—since if this were not the case, there would be no conflict. It is obviously necessary to be completely clear in your own mind what those symptoms/emotions are before commencing this type of therapy.)

"Take some time now and listen to what the part on the left has to say about what she feels. And repeat to me everything that is being said—but I want you to be uncritical. You see she has a reason to have those thoughts and feelings."

Wait for response.

"Now turn towards the part on your right... and take some time to listen to what the part on the right has to say about what she thinks and feels. And once more repeat to me everything that is being said."

Wait for response.

"Be aware as you are hearing and seeing that each has a point... and perhaps it is time now to see how each part reached this pattern of thought and feelings and the purpose which each was serving. Create directly in front of you a large screen—sort of like a cinema screen...

Now let each part show you when and why she developed this particular feeling or thought. Start with the part on the left and tell me what is being shown to you.

"It could be something recent or something which occurred many years ago. I don't know what it is that you are going to be shown."

Wait for response.

"Now do the same with the part on the right. Good."

Wait for response.

"Thank each part for sharing with us her experience. I would like you now to ask both parts whether they agree that while they both have a right to their thoughts and feelings about this conflict, both are suffering?"

Wait for response.

"Do both parts agree that a consensus must be reached in order to allow both to achieve her goals?"

Wait for response.

"Now I'd like you to take some time and—using all your wisdom, all your knowledge, all your understanding—suggest a solution which will enable each to live in harmony within you. Take your time and if you need my help just let me know."

It is not always necessary to know what the compromise is but it is important that all parts present must reach total agreement, and embrace and reintegrate as one.

Case study

Now follows a full account by a client, himself a counsellor, who experienced this technique and whom we thank for permitting us to reproduce it here.

The client had a weight problem. He had just invited the different parts or sub-personalities of himself to come in and sit round the table. When one side came in, he was furious. His main statement was:

Client X: I want it and I want it now!

This he demanded in a barely-controlled, hate-filled and furious way, through tight lips and held breath. It was implicit that he would not enter into any negotiation. His second statement was held with all the intensity of the first:

Client X: I am not going to miss out!

When the therapist invited the other part to sit opposite the angry part, the angry part went berserk.

Therapist: Why does he feel like this?

Client X: I just cannot stand the way he is.

Therapist: Can you say more about how he is, what he does that makes you so furious?

Client X: He comes in and presents…

There was a pause while the client tried desperately to get his feelings into words. This was a struggle with the intensity of his feelings before putting them into words. He needed encouragement. He was slipping into despair and the therapist sensed this.

Therapist: It's okay, take your time.

Then it just tumbled out of the client.

Client X: He presents himself as so good, so enduring. Then, see, that's what he does—hypes up all the anxiety and doubt.

The therapist gave more encouragement.

Therapist: Go on. It seems like you have a point.

Client X: Well, when he does that I can have no peace.

Therapist: Does he do anything else?

Client X: Yes, he makes me feel this raw, uncomfortable rage at his lack of trust, only food calms me down.

The client felt amazed and bewildered at the insight. It is essential that the therapist maintains a sympathetic and supportive attitude under these and similar circumstances.

Therapist: Can you go on?

Client X: If I don't get the food, I feel I am deprived, missing out, cheated, I must have it to calm the raw, uncomfortable rage.

Therapist: Okay, just have a rest, be with all that a while.

The client was grateful. He needed time to integrate all this. After a few moments, the therapist continued:

Therapist: I want you to ask the other side what he feels. Do you think you could you do that?

Client X: Yes.

The angry side asked grudgingly:

Client X: What do you feel?

Client Y: Well, I am the good, enduring, patient side.

After a pause the therapist moved in and asked:

Therapist: Can you say more, what do you do?

Client Y: I let in trust and only expect the negative. To protect (name) from being hurt, shocked. So if I don't trust the good or let it in, then (name) can't be taken by surprise, tricked.

Therapist *(after a moment or two): Why would (name) be hurt by being open to the good?*

Client Y: *He would be completely vulnerable.*

Therapist: *Is there anything else you do?*

Client Y: *I fuel him with doubt and anxiety so he won't trust.*

The client was clearly shocked at these realisations. As he integrated this new information, quite an amazing shift in thought processes was going on as he came to a fuller realisation of the machinations of this part of his psyche. The unconscious defence-mechanisms had impacted on his whole life up to this point.

The session was approaching an end but the therapist thought it vital to initiate some repair dialogue between the two parts if possible. He asked the furious part:

Therapist: *What could the good, enduring part do that would help you?*

Client X: *Tell him that if you could just start to let in some good, some compliments, have some trust, it would so nourish me instead of filling me up on a diet of distrust, anxiety and doubt.*

Client Y: *I'll try.*

The enduring part still was reeling from the realisation of his damaging defence-strategy and the therapist quietly ended the session. The client was later to report his growing awareness that it was a defence-strategy which had gone wrong, saying: "It was doing more harm than good. More harm, in fact, than what it was supposed to be protecting me from."

Finally and crucially at another session the client said:

Client: *I dare not believe I have found the answer to my weight problem, after all this time. I desperately don't want to be disappointed by another false dawn.*

Almost immediately, there was a sudden awareness:

> **Client:** *And that's it, isn't it? The very self-defeating mechanism working again for the best intentions but preventing me from believing and trusting that something really is healing for me.*

Table-Top Therapy™ is an extremely versatile tool to use with clients who have a high need for control. One of its greatest features is that it affords the client the ability to enter a selective-thinking mode, and therefore is a subtle introduction to the feeling of hypnosis without the word ever being mentioned.

Chapter 20

The Repeater—Dealing with Negative Programming

Often with clients who suffer anxiety or other kinds of nervousness you will notice a particular phrase or word being used over and above its intended or normal use. It is as if the client's unconscious mind is holding on to a catch-word or catch-phrase and repeating it over and over again.

These phrases tend to be negative and are most often used inappropriately as a defence in the client's present life. However, such phrases can be an excellent source of uncovering repressed material from the client.

Here are a few examples of this phenomenon:

A client, from the point of arrival at your consulting room, will apologise: for being early by two minutes; for walking in or sitting down before you; or even if you make a mistake by asking the client to sit in one place and then correct yourself. In fact, it seems that every move is followed by: "I'm sorry."

At first you may think that this is a very polite client. Or that he is just a little nervous. A second example is of a client who precedes his response with: "I don't know." All too often he will give an answer like: "I don't know, but I should be able to make my next appointment" or "I don't know, I'll try to relax."

At first this client may give the impression of being quite resistant to the therapy until you begin to realise the frequency of his response. The technique shown here to assist in the uncovering of the neuroses in these instances is simple to use, requires very little visualisation and can be applied quickly.

Repeater script

Use a physical, progressive relaxation technique of your choice to allow the client to become as detached as possible and then proceed as follows:

"Now place your awareness in the darkness of your mind, and as you place your awareness in the darkness of your mind, I want you to set aside all your everyday thoughts…because now you don't have to do anything, you don't even have to think about what I'm going to say to you or even what I'm going to ask you to think about…

"All I want you to do while you relax there, with your breathing calm and peaceful, just listening to the sound of my voice, is to see a word. You may wonder what the word is which I'm going to tell you. Well, that's okay. And it doesn't matter how you see this word… it could be written in ink, black or blue on white paper or it could be written in chalk, perhaps even white chalk, on a blackboard. Like on a blackboard on the inside of your mind and the word I'm going to ask you to see is the word: SORRY.

"That's right, the word SORRY, and the more you see the word SORRY, the clearer it becomes, the brighter it becomes and the larger it becomes. Just focus on the word SORRY more and more, that's right. And notice how it is written, perhaps in capitals or perhaps very tiny print. Notice the colour of the letters—perhaps they are all the same or perhaps they are all different. Just focus on that word, the word SORRY. It's like a magnet drawing your attention to it, and as you do become more and more drawn to the word SORRY, the clearer it becomes. The clearer it becomes to you, the larger it becomes.

"Feel it as every muscle, fibre and tissue of your body experiences the word SORRY, every cell within your body repeating that word SORRY. And the more you focus, the brighter it becomes and the more it fills your whole body until your body is vibrating with the word SORRY. Every part of you, your legs SORRY, your arms SORRY, your chest SORRY, your head SORRY, SORRY, SORRY, SORRY. Your feet SORRY, your tummy SORRY, your hands SORRY. Until you are bursting with SORRY.

"Now hear the word SORRY in your mind, in your thoughts, hear it getting louder and louder and louder, until it feels like it will explode out of every pore of your skin, just hear that word SORRY, SORRY, SORRY circulating all through your body. SORRY, SORRY, SORRY bouncing and ricocheting off the inside walls of yourself. Hear SORRY echoing in your ears SORRY, SORRY, SORRY.

"Repeat it to yourself SORRY, SORRY, SORRY—that's right—keep going SORRY, SORRY, SORRY, SORRY over and over again repeating it in your mind. And now I want you to actually say the word SORRY. Say it out loud, say it right now, yes, right now, say it, say the word SORRY. And again. And again, go on, keep repeating the word SORRY, SORRY, SORRY, SORRY—that's right—every cell of you screaming out the word SORRY—your entire body seeing, hearing, feeling SORRY.

"On the count of three find yourself in another place, another time with that thought, that feeling… one, two, three. Where are you?"

Examples

Here are some examples of where the client might find himself:

"I'm sorry"

Client: *I'm looking at the carpet.*

Therapist: *What carpet?*

Client: *The one in the lounge.*

Therapist: *What do you hear?*

Client: *I'm saying: "I'M SORRY, I'M SORRY."*

Therapist: *Why are you sorry?*

Client: *If I say I'M SORRY, he might not hit me.*

Therapist: *Who might not hit you?*

> *Client: My Dad. I'M SORRY. He's walking towards me taking his belt off. I don't know what I've done. I'M SORRY. Don't hit me. I'M SORRY. If I say I'M SORRY enough, he might not hit me.*

"I don't know"

The father of the client in this next example was a very violent person and the fear which had been instilled in the client was overwhelming.

> *Client: I'm sitting at the table doing my homework.*
>
> *Therapist: What happens next?*
>
> *Client: Dad comes in and asks me: "Where's Mum?" I DON'T KNOW. "Where's your sister?" I DON'T KNOW. "You don't know anything. You're not fucking anything. You don't know, you don't know anything, do you, eh?" I DON'T KNOW.*

This technique can also be used for your compulsive disorder clients. A female client constantly outlined everything visually— the squares on the carpet, the squares within the squares on the carpet, the carpet, the lamp, the flower-pot, the therapist. She would just sit and visually outline everything. So instead of I'M SORRY or I DON'T KNOW, STUCK OUTLINING was used. On the count of 'three' she was in a lobby looking at Dad coming down the stairs towards the front door.

> *Client: It's a bright sunny day.*
>
> *Therapist: How do you know it's a bright sunny day?*
>
> *Client: I can see the sun shining in the front porch, it's shining right through. I can only see his outline.*

The client abreacted as she remembered that this was the last time she had seen him alive.

Whilst not to be considered as a replacement for analytical therapy, this technique can provide rapid relief for a great number of anxiety symptoms associated with negativity.

Chapter 21

Symbolic Removal of Symptoms

The symbolic removal of symptoms in order to the find their cause is a very useful and powerful way to reduce a client's resistance to the trance experience. There are plenty of techniques readily available to help clients to *dispose* of their symptoms. This does not always bring about a satisfactory and permanent solution to the problem, as one is uncertain how/when any new symptom will manifest itself via the process of symptom substitution. This technique is rather like a pinpoint analysis, in that it is principally designed to deal with one specific problem. It is also an appropriate technique for use with hypnophobic clients. **Symbolic removal** is best described as *the removal of symptoms to make way for the revelation of the cause.*

Overview of the therapy

Occasionally a client's symptoms are clear and obvious and can be isolated and even given a reasonably physical explanation. Typically, a client may come complaining of a persistent pain in the neck, pain in the shoulder or tummy pain when at an interview.

Of course, not all pain is psychosomatic, so you should be sure that before you start any form of therapy that the client has sought medical advice first. Also ensure that it is something which has been with the client for some time. In other words that the client did not fall the week before and damage herself.

On the basis that the pain or discomfort has been persistent and no medical or logical explanation can be found, then it would be reasonable to assume that the symptom is a message from the unconscious mind that something is wrong. The reason why it is there is that on some level the client is resisting some element of her truth or is being protected from the pain of an old event. The neurosis is making itself heard and felt in whatever way it can by taking the path of least resistance.

What this form of therapy does, through the appropriate use of questions, is to put the client in a position to enter into the language and mode of communication of her own unconscious mind. Using the client's imagination, she will gently drift from the real world and the symptom into the trance-world seeking the cause. You will help bring about a symbolic removal of the symptom and then bring forward the cause as if it would appear to have no function or purpose left.

To begin with, you need to clearly define what the client wants to happen. This will also help to reduce the possibility of any secondary gains or hidden agendas. A good and powerful question using 'clean language' would be:

What do you want to happen here?

What do you want?

There are 3 possible responses to such a question and each has a value in therapy:

(1) the client may say what she wants

(2) the client may say what she does not want

(3) the client may say she does not know

Although eliciting as much information as possible is vital to the therapy, information gathering should be achieved with the least amount of suggestion. Also, it is advisable that the language used fits the client's understanding. In the following examples you will see that the less said, the more the client enters into her own unconscious language and deepens the trance.

There are several ways a client may present her problem. It may be a physical sensation which she experiences at a particular time or situation. Or it may be that she lacks an ability to express herself or to perform in given situations. It makes little difference which way the problem is presented, as by a process of elimination you will inevitably conclude that she has a physical effect. Let us now assume that the client says she knows what she wants—for example:

> **Client:** *I want to feel confident—and not anxious—at work.*

The next step would be to establish how the client perceives confidence. Therefore, ask your client to tell you what she would see herself doing if she were to have confidence—that is, an outcome with confidence. Simple questions which would help the client would be:

> **Therapist:** *What do you see yourself doing when you have confidence? What do you hear yourself saying when you have confidence?*

Eliciting information from your client can take some time—be patient and allow this time. This will help your client to enter into deeper trance. Gaining the client's epistemology of want through questions will help to further reduce resistance.

Suggested questions:

> *"And when you have confidence, what is that like?"*

> *"How do you know that you know that you want confidence?"*

> *"How long have you known that you have wanted it?"*

> *"Has there been a time when you knew you did not want it?"*

The object here is to define the client's want into a clear, achievable goal for therapy. Becoming more aware of the client's language will give you insight into how the client uses language to describe experiences and inner realities and will help you to establish her own internal modus operandi. This will help you later on when uncovering-therapy commences.

There are principally four ways in which the client will communicate with you and we will outline briefly what they are:

Memory

"If only I could have said that to my boss last week, then ..."

Symbolic

"My boss is a pain in the neck."

Metaphors

"Speaking to the boss is hard, it's like there's a brick wall."

Semantics

"It's so difficult talking to the boss, he's so boring, he should smarten himself up."

Through the understanding which we gain, we are able to establish whether her need is achievable in therapy and whether we can test the want or the outcome. Sometimes just doing this, in itself, can bring about the client's desired outcome. It is not our concern what might be a desirable outcome for the client, all we are concerned with—at any time—is testing that the want is a belief which is strongly held. That is, can it be altered in any way? Are there any alternatives? It is only then that we can proceed with a therapeutic intervention which will help the client to achieve what she wants. So now let us sum up at this time what you will have achieved by listening to your client:

(1) an understanding of the client's desired outcome

(2) the current situation for the client

(3) the client's internal language

With this information you are ready to proceed to the next phase of isolating the symptom and giving the symptom an identity of its own—in effect dissociating it from the client.

Case study 1

Below are excerpts from a session with a client who suffered from anxiety attacks. When he was in an office with other people he found himself with a sense of being enclosed. The anxiety, we established early on, was in his stomach area.

> **Therapist:** *And when that anxious feeling is there what happens?*

The client described the symptoms of panic from a cold sweat to jelly legs.

> **Therapist:** *And how do you know when that panic feeling is coming?*

> **Client:** *I get that feeling in my stomach.*

The client pointed to his solar plexus.

> **Therapist:** *Tell me about that feeling.*

The client began to describe the feeling in his stomach as being a frightened feeling. At this point we asked the client to look inwardly as if he could see inside himself, and we asked him to describe what it was that he saw. We were aiming to give this feeling an identity.

It is okay at this point to ask the client to imagine or to pretend that he can see what it is that he is experiencing inside. For example, to identify where that feeling is or whether it is lighter or darker than where that feeling is not.

> **Client:** *It's lighter.*

> **Therapist:** *And if it had a colour what sort of colour would it have?*

> **Client:** *Like a sort of green.*

> **Therapist:** *And when you look at that sort of green, so that I can see it too, imagine it's more like a shape—liken it to something.*

163

Client: *It's like a tube.*

Therapist: *And when you look at green tube what sort of size is green tube?*

The client indicated with his hands an approximate area of about 6 to 10 inches and about an inch in diameter.

Therapist: *When you look at green tube that's about that size, can you tell me if it's the same colour all the way round?*

Client: *Yes, it is green everywhere.*

Therapist: *Without getting too close to it and disturbing it, what else can you tell me about green tube?*

Client: *Well, actually, it's not a tube, it's more like a rod.*

Therapist: *That's good. And as you look at rod now, can you tell me, if you could touch green rod, what sort of texture would it have?*

Client: *Sort of smooth like metal.*

Therapist: *So, as you look at rod that's green and sort of smooth like metal, if you could feel its temperature, what sort of temperature would rod have?*

Client: *Cold.*

Therapist: *And as you look at rod, green and sort of smooth and cold, if you could hear rod, what sound do you imagine rod makes?*

Client: *None.*

Therapist: *If you could look right inside rod what else would you see?*

Client: *It's just solid.*

Therapist: *As you look round about rod, do you see rod connected to anything else?*

Client: No.

Therapist: Now as you look at rod that's green and sort of smooth and cold, I would like you to allow your imagination here to help you to imagine a way which will move that rod from in there to out here. Now take as long as you need to do this.

The client took about three minutes to respond. Sometimes it can take longer. On one occasion it was fifteen minutes before the client had thought of a way. Occasionally a client will say that there is nothing that will remove it, when you will need to intervene—as little as possible—to suggest ways that *you* think would work until something feels right to the client. There is a very powerful method shown later in this chapter.

Client: I've got to cut it out.

Therapist: You're going to cut it out. Have you got everything you need to cut it out?

Client: Yes. I'm going to use a scalpel.

Therapist: Before you start, what I would like you to do is to put on some special gloves so that rod is not disturbed when you bring rod out. And when you have rod out, let me know. Is that okay?

Client: Yes.

Several minutes elapsed before the client started to speak.

Client: I've got it out.

Therapist: That's good. Now place rod on the floor while we think about what we're going to do next. Because, you see, what needs to happen for you to be free of rod is that we find a way to totally destroy rod so that rod can never return. So as I speak to you I do know that the right idea will come to you from your unconscious mind. Now take some time and tell me what would need to happen to rod so that rod is no longer.

Client: I suppose I could melt it.

Therapist: And when you think about melting rod what comes to mind?

Client: One of those things that the Terminator jumped in like a boiling, molten metal.

Therapist: That's a good idea. Imagine as you stand looking down at one of those huge vats full of smelting metal, what's going to happen to rod?

Client: It's going to disintegrate.

Therapist: That's right. Let me know when you are satisfied that rod is completely destroyed

Client: Yes, that's it, it's gone.

Therapist: Great, well done. How does it feel now that rod is no longer where rod used to be? More importantly, look and tell me what has taken rod's place.

Client: It's like all the rest now. It's like a dark red, it feels okay.

Therapist: Would you like to know what rod was doing there in the first place?

Client: Yes.

Therapist: When you next hear the number 3 you'll find yourself at the very moment that rod first came. 1, 2, 3. Where do you find yourself?

Before asking the above question look for REM (Rapid Eye Movement) in your client.

Client: I can't get out, they're fighting on the floor, I can't get out, I can't get the bolt to come down. I can't reach high enough to pull it down. There's blood all over the floor. My Dad's lying on the floor. There's blood everywhere. My Uncle's just smashed a sheet of glass on my Dad's head.

Therapist: Go on.

Client: I'm scared.

Therapist: Where are you scared?

Client: By the door.

Therapist: What's happening now?

Client: I want to get some help but I can't get out.

Therapist: Why can't you get out?

Client: I can't reach high enough to pull the bolt down.

Therapist: What bolt?

Client: The bolt at the top of the garage door. I can't reach it.

Therapist: Tell me what happens next?

Client: My Uncle's running towards the garage doors. He's opened the doors and he's gone out. I don't know what to do. I can't move. I don't know what to do. I think he's dead.

Therapist: And what happens next.

Client: I've gone to get my Mum.

The client in this case was aged about ten or eleven at the time of the incident and had witnessed a fight between his uncle and his father in which his uncle, after an argument, smashed a sheet of glass over his father's head. The client then managed to run out and, unable to find his Mum, told a neighbour who called an ambulance. The father eventually recovered.

This is a very simple example but it probably reflects 80% of those clients with whom this form of therapy is used. In this case the rod represented the bolt which was green and cold on the garage doors. The panic/anxiety attack which the client experienced was at his own inability to leave and, therefore, left him with a feeling of being trapped until the uncle opened the door.

Probably the most important point which we need to make in the initial stages of enquiry is the vital importance of giving the symptom a significance or personality. It is as if the client no longer sees it as part of him. The importance of symbolically destroying the feeling or personality is a crucial part of the therapy.

Case study 2

This case is interesting for the fact that the client was adamantly opposed to any form of hypnosis. She presented for therapy after experiencing panic attacks in supermarkets and large stores; the problem had started when her son was about three years old. It soon became obvious that she was very frightened and suspicious; she almost immediately stated that under no circumstances did she want anyone to hypnotise her. After being assured that there was a very powerful and efficient technique that could be used without any need for her to go into a trance state, she made an appointment for the following week. Even though she had been assured that there would be no need for trance, she was in a highly nervous state when she arrived in the therapist's office.

She was asked to describe—through a second by second account—the lead up to a panic attack in any situation of her choice. She was soon describing virtually a full panic attack from the jelly legs to the perspiration, and again insisting that she did not want to go into hypnosis as it frightened her. She accepted the assurance that there was no need to go into a trance, especially when it was mentioned that she could keep her eyes open for as long as she liked or close them if she would like them to be more comfortable. Immediately after this, she was asked where the feeling first starts.

Client: It feels like it's in my tummy.

Therapist: And I wonder if you could imagine as you look at that area of your body, knowing that that's where the feeling starts, whether it's the same or it's different from the rest of your body?

Client: It's different.

Therapist: And when you look at that different area, how large an area is that different area?

Client: This might sound silly but it's bigger than I am.

Therapist: That's right. Sometimes it is. But I'd like you to be of a little more help to me. Is that okay?

Client: Yes.

Therapist: What I'd like you to do—as you look down into that different area—is to tell me does it have a different colour?

Client: Yes, it does.

Therapist: What colour is it?

Client: It's brown.

Therapist: And if you could—so that I can see it in my mind's eye— give it a shape, what sort of shape would it have?

Client: It's like a box.

Therapist: And when you look at box what can you tell me about box?

Client: Well, it's strange because it's a sort of cardboard box, the type which you fold up. But it has not been folded, so it looks as if you could look through it.

At this point we went though all the different elements—texture, temperature, sound, colour of inside, etc. By now, she had closed her eyes but when she was asked if she would like to find a way to remove box, her eyes immediately snapped open. Then:

Client: (screams) No, I can't do that.

Therapist: That's fine. That's okay. You really don't have to do anything you don't want to do. How about—if only just for a while—taking box out and putting it right down there by your legs so that we can do the work that we need to do and then you can choose to keep box or to let box go. Is that all right with you?

Client: Okay. But I don't want to let it go.

Therapist: Now that you are comfortable and box is by your legs, just have a look and tell me what's in place of box now?

Client: Nothing. It's just black.

Therapist: That's good. With black now in place how would it feel if you were to go into a supermarket?

Client: That's okay now.

Therapist: Would you like to know what purpose box served there in your tummy?

Client: No.

Therapist: So you don't mind if box comes back?

Client: Yes, I do.

Therapist: All that needs to happen is to let box tell you something which box has been wanting to tell you for a long time. And once you know the thing that you've been looking to understand about how you've been feeling, then would you need to have that feeling again? Or would you rather keep box?

Client: No.

Therapist: Good. When you next hear the number 3 you'll imagine yourself somewhere else and without thinking about why you are somewhere else tell me where it is that you find yourself. 1, 2, 3. Tell me where you find yourself.

At this point client vigorously protested:

Client: No, this can't be happening. I'm just imagining it. This isn't real.

Therapist: What isn't real?

Client: No, this can't be happening. I can't believe it!

After some gentle manoeuvring the client began to reveal that she was aged between three and four in a hotel room and while her mother was out her father was sexually abusing her orally. She recalled in great detail the bedspread's colour and design. The session ended with her being totally convinced that this was all a false-memory syndrome and just a figment of her imagination.

She was then asked whether she would like to put the box back or to leave it in the therapist's care until the following week. She agreed to leave it in the safe-keeping of the therapist.

On her return she had investigated some of the details and discovered to her disappointment that the place which she had recalled really did exist. Her mother vaguely remembered that particular holiday to the seaside. Over the next three sessions, the full extent of the abuse was gradually revealed. It gave her a great insight into her behaviour including remembering one occasion, when she was aged approximately ten years, having a compelling desire to touch a baby cousin's genitals and the only way in which she could deal with it was to run out of the house.

Now you are probably wondering what the box represented. Her father ran a garment factory and in the factory there were hundreds of these boxes stored and she used to see them continually when she worked there as a teenager. She even recalled a scene in which her father was shouting at her to work faster while packing a box.

Occasionally the symptom is represented in two places—in, say, the tummy and in the head, for example:

Client: When I walk into the canteen I get this pain in my neck and my tummy rumbles and then tightens up.

Deal with each symptom separately, even if they are simultaneously triggered. When the symptoms have all been destroyed, only then should you ask the question: *"Would you like to know what purpose they served?"*

With some clients you may find that they cannot imagine a way in which to get rid of the symptom after they have created a visual and/or physical representation of it. In these cases the following suggestion, or any derivation of it, is very useful:

> *"That's fine. I want you to imagine that down here by my side, there on the floor, I have a box, a metal box, a metal box which is lead-lined. And this lead-lined metal box has a slam-shut lid that locks. And I want you to take your time now and take X and place it in the box. When it is in the box I want you to tell me that it is in the box, and then I will shut the lid down and you can continue as if it cannot return."*

Chapter 22

Using Your Client's Symptoms

When a client first presents himself to you for therapy, it is odds-on that he has spent a fair amount of time attempting to ignore his symptoms or to develop a pattern of avoidance behaviour of sorts. In this chapter, we are going to help him to do exactly the opposite, and in so doing, to gain an understanding and subsequent release.

This is actually a lot easier than it sounds, since we will be exploring thought processes which are totally unfamiliar to the client and to which he therefore has no 'ready-made' resistance patterns in existence. Also, for the same reason, there will be few, if any, preconceived ideas or concepts to hinder us in our endeavours. In other words, the client will be more co-operative because he will not have been down this particular road before and will not have applied intellectual effort that can get in our way.

This method has three particular advantages over some other forms of 'uncovering' or regression/analytical work:

(1) It needs no formal hypnotic induction, though most clients will drift into hypnosis as we work with them, heightening their awareness.

(2) It is faster than 'standard' analytical techniques where conditioned response or cumulative trauma is concerned.

(3) It is more effective with the logical/analytical type of client than are some other techniques, since it works in a chronological (rather than free-association) manner and actually *employs* their natural tendency to self-analyse.

It does have one drawback, in that it can come to an abrupt halt where true repression exists. In practice, though, this is not a huge problem, since you would then employ hypnosis and regression/analytical techniques to release it, using the information you have already gathered as a starting-point.

We will be working with the idea in mind that there is always a purpose for the existence of a symptom pattern; it is 'designed' to somehow protect the client's psyche from situations or concepts which the subconscious perceives as harmful, even mortally dangerous. So, little by little, we are going to guide our client gently back along the track he has followed from the moment the need for that symptom pattern came into being, until we find the source.

We must not forget that the original symptom may have been substituted many times and may have taken on a 'format' calculated to totally divert attention from the original neurosis, especially in the case of guilt complex. In this way, what started out as masturbatory guilt, for example, can end up years later as an obsessive need to recheck locks and switches, a crippling 'neediness' for partners, anxiety about eating in public, a fear of heights, kleptomania, claustrophobia... or even all of these, and more, in succession. Usually, the client will be unaware of the process of symptom substitution and may not even be aware that he has ever had a psychological problem other than his currently presenting one. As irrational and unlikely as it may seem, the need to disguise the neurotic drive discourages awareness of change in the way that it is expressed—as far as your client is concerned, it has always been a matter of 'just the way I am'. He may well express surprise to realise that he was once inclined towards depression, for example.

Much of the rest of this chapter is written in the form of dialogue with the client, since it is by far the easiest way for you to understand how and why it works. Notice that the therapist's language is as clean as it possibly can be.

Your client preparation talk should be similar to that which you would use for a client about to undergo analysis, outlining the idea of expectation and belief systems, conditioned response, the 'invisibility' of the sub-conscious, etc. If you mention repression, do so very lightly. A good method here is to say something like: *"Now, we're not actually going to be searching for buried memories as such, because, most of the time, they've simply been forgotten rather than repressed. But, of course, if there is anything there that needs to be found we'll certainly find it."*

Starting work

Essentially, we are going to use a form of regression therapy and this will become apparent to you; it will also become apparent, as we begin to 'home in' on the problem, that there are a few very important differences.

If you have decided to use hypnosis with this particular client, then it is probably a good idea, in the first session, to use one of the 'subconscious primer' techniques that can be found in Chapters Four to Six. Then the second and any subsequent sessions can follow a similar format to that shown here. For the moment, we will assume that you are working without formal hypnosis, although you will suggest to your client that he close his eyes; if he wishes not to, you can still work but there are likely to be more attempts at resistance.

You can be facing or sitting adjacent to your client but you need to be able to observe body language (see Chapter Eleven) and face expression. When you are ready, begin:

> *"All right, good, you just make yourself comfortable in that chair now... all right?... Now, it's probably slightly easier for you to concentrate if you allow your eyes to close, but whatever feels best to you, just do that... that's right... and perhaps allow your breathing to steady for a moment or two... yes... that's good... and let your body be as lazy as you want it to be... good... now, I'd like you to think of...(draw attention to the symptom pattern)... for a moment or two. Don't worry if you feel a little uncomfortable as you do so, because that's all quite normal and is actually a very good sign...that's right...I wonder if you would now let your mind just drift back a while to the first time you can remember feeling like that... it doesn't matter if that's last week, last year, or some time before that... your mind knows just where to go... just take your time and let your thoughts search out that first time when you learnt you could feel like that... when you find it, just tell me what you find yourself with..."*

Here, you will wait for a few moments while your client searches in whichever mode is best for them. At this point there is no need for any pressure, since we are simply attempting to find out whether we are dealing with a substitute or primary symptom. If there is no response after two minutes or so, then probe gently. All the time, watch for signs of emotional response; in addition to those given in Chapter Eleven, these might be: a sudden increase in facial flush, especially across/near the bridge of the nose; increased respiration or drawing of breath; eyes opening or closing; a movement as if about to speak; change in facial expression (which may be very subtle). If you see *any* of these for more than a moment, there is almost certainly some emotional work going on. At that point, you would invite the client to tell you exactly what was in their thoughts. Of course, if you were working in an Ericksonian manner you might commence here with: *"That's right..."* then continue as you perceive best. But you will still need to establish how old the client is in this moment of his history, since we need to get his thoughts back to the *original* symptom, which is usually present during the childhood years, even though it may not be evident as a symptom.

Case study

We will continue with part of a case history to illustrate more clearly how and why this method works. The client was 42, a successful, very down-to-earth businessman, with a stomach problem which became acute when he perceived that he was under pressure. At the hospital, the endoscopy had shown nothing more than a mild inflammation of the stomach lining and not the smallest indicator of an ulcer, even though he frequently suffered severe heartburn. When he presented to the consulting room, he had just returned from a two-week holiday abroad, during which time there had been no real problem. He was now back at work and already beginning to find the familiar sensation of acid surging into the oesophagus when he felt under pressure. We will pick it up after he had allowed his thoughts to drift back for about a minute or so. The dotted lines show where there was relatively inconsequential conversation which has been deleted.

> **Client:** *"I'm remembering one of the first times I felt this gut trouble... I'm about 30, I think."*

> **Therapist:** *Good... tell me about that.*

Client: *Not a lot to tell, really...I'm just remembering it hurting. Don't know where I was, though.*

Therapist: *And when was it the right time for it to hurt you?*

Client: *It wasn't! I never wanted it to!*

Therapist: *But when was it the right time for **IT** to hurt you?*

This is where we depart from 'normal' regression work, actually giving the symptom a reason to exist and permission to affect.

Client: *Oh, I see... well, I remember once when I was out with the boys. We were playing darts and I hadn't played much before so I started losing, really badly. I **hate** losing, really can't stand the embarrassment. They all started taking the piss and that set my gut off.*

It is necessary to recall an actual event for the symptom we are working with, for the chronological location. It would seem likely that this was a substitute symptom, so we probe.

Therapist: *And that was one of the first times anything had set your gut off...*

Client: *I think so, yes...*

Therapist: *And when it wasn't setting your gut off... what was it doing then?*

Most times, your client will accept without noticing that you are now talking about an 'it' that has been doing something else before it started 'performing' his current symptom. If the client had asked what that meant, the therapist would have said: "Pressure", since that was the circumstance under which he became acutely aware of his symptom.

Client: *Nothing... I can't think of anything...*

Therapist: *Tell me what your life was like, back then in those days.*

We would offer encouragement and interaction here, just a conversation about the sort of things that your client has already told you causes difficulty. In this case, the conversation could include work (since that was what had brought him to therapy in the first place), pressure (for the same reason), interaction with peers and opposite/preferred sex relationships.

…

> *Client: Now I'm remembering meeting my wife and taking her out for the first time.*

> *Therapist: How does that feel?*

> *Client: Good… actually, I remember I used to have a bit of trouble eating in front of people sometimes. I took her out for a meal. It was uncomfortable.*

This, of course, is what we are looking for—the symptom before the current one, even though it had not really been noticed by the client as a symptom as such.

> *Therapist: And it was right for uncomfortable to be there, because…?*

Always ignore grammar when 'feeding back'. Again, the symptom is being treated as an entity—the effective question was not: "Why did you feel uncomfortable?" but: "Why did that uncomfortable want to be there?"

> *Client: Well, it was just a bit of awkwardness 'cos I wasn't used to going to the places she wanted to go in. I liked cafes. She liked poofy restaurants.*

> *Therapist: And how did you learn that those restaurants were poofy?*

> *Client: Just thought they were. My mum always said they were.*

Here, there was a sudden foot waggle, showing discomfort and a possibly unadmitted thought.

Therapist: But your wife liked them.

Client: Yeh. Still does.

Therapist: And do you still think they're poofy?

There is a need to fully explore each successive symptom as we move back, in order to trigger the subconscious thought processes to the next.

Client: Um... yeh, I do really. I quite like em now, though. My wife is right—it's great to go and get really looked after.

Therapist: What does Mum think about you going to those places now?

Client: Dunno. I don't tell her.

Again, there was the foot waggle; he was obviously uncomfortable about Mum in some way. Plus, of course, he was not letting her know he went into 'poofy' restaurants. She still had an active influence on his psyche. Here, we might ask: "Because...?"

...

Client: Actually, here's a funny thing... I've suddenly flipped right back to when I was about 17.

Therapist: Tell me.

*Client: Oh, it's just the first time I stayed out really late. I was round my friend's house and my mother suddenly turned up at his front door. She was crying and saying she thought I'd been killed. It was **really** embarrassing.*

More foot waggling.

Therapist: And embarrassing wanted to be there, because...?

Client: I dunno. 'Cos Mum was, I suppose.

This sort of response almost certainly links his symptom to his mother.

> **Therapist:** *What else was there about that time?*

There had to be something else, because, apart from the clue of the foot waggling, his mind had gone to another uncomfortable moment. The previous symptom had to be somewhere close! The rest of that session, though, drew a complete blank. The client's subconscious had decided not to play the game any more that day.

Oscillation

The next two sessions covered similar ground, with the client's mind going backwards and forwards between current and 17 years old or so. This 'oscillation' effect is not unusual; it is as though the subconscious *needs* to explore several different facets of the problem. We should just go along with that all the time new material is being recalled. The client began to realise that he had had indicators of anxiety far earlier than he had thought, but it was his third session before we found recognisable symptoms from his teen years.

> **Client:** *I'd forgotten all about this...I remember I went through a stage of blushing when I tried to talk to girls. I had to pretend I wasn't interested, else all my mates'd've seen it... I think I sorta got a grip on it. About 16, I was. But I used to get a sort of knot in my stomach for ages after that.*

> **Therapist:** *That's right...a knot in the stomach.*

More foot waggling occurred quite sharply.

> **Therapist:** *What are you thinking right now?*

> **Client:** *Um... I just remembered the rash I used to get. Mum said it was nervous eczema or something.*

> **Therapist:** *And that nervous eczema wanted to be there, because...?*

> **Client:** *It used to flare up when I was pissed off with school.*

So here we are back in the formative years with a 'nervous' symptom! But it still may not be the originating one, so we still carry on checking.

Therapist: *Can your mind go to the first time it flared up?*

Client: *Yeh... I think so...It was school sports day and I couldn't take part, 'cos I was covered with it. Actually, I've just this second realised it was exactly a year after the sack race. I'm 9.*

This is a spontaneous regression to a year before, so we capitalise on it, especially since there was an attempt not to 'go back', via the 'I'm 9' statement.

Therapist: *Tell me about that sack race.*

Client: *Oh, yeh... I remember that all right...*

His complexion became quite dark and his body language stopped completely. Spontaneous hypnosis was occurring, and the therapist said nothing, waiting.

Client: *It was sports day and Mum was there... she's not normal, my mum. Never bloody was. So embarrassing.*

Therapist: *Tell me about that.*

Client: *Well, all the other kids' parents were just clapping and stuff...* (He screwed his face up and complained that his stomach was 'in a right bloody knot', indicating that we were right on it now). *"She has to jump up and down like a bleeding lunatic! Shrieking my name over and again... c'mon Ronnie! C'mon Ronnie! Ronnie! Ronnie! I got a right panic. D'you know what? I can actually **feel** it right now, just like I was there.*

Therapist: *That's right! You can feel it, just like you were there!*

Client: *It was the bloody sack race, so I've got this sack all round my legs and I got in such a state with her yelling at me, I tried to bleeding well run instead of jump!*

Therapist: *And you tried to run...*

Client: *I fell right on my bloody face, didn't I? Everybody's started laughing and I was **really** embarrassed.* (He put both his hands up to his head and grimaced.) *She's yelling at me to get up... and every time I did I was in such a state I tried to run again. I could see all these other kids getting away from me and what with her bloody well yelling and shrieking my name over and again I had no chance... So I was last. I could feel myself going as red as a beetroot and I threw the sack away and ran off the bloody field as fast as I could. Everybody was laughing their heads off and **she** was **still** yelling out Ronnie! Ronnie! I just wanted to **die** with bloody embarrassment.*

This proved to be the first link in a cumulative trauma chain which had been initiated and perpetuated by the client's mother's 'over the top' behaviour. He had some difficulty in recognising how such a relatively unimportant event (to the adult mind) could have had such a profound effect upon him but the next time he came to see me, he was delighted to tell me his stomach had felt calm the entire week. We investigated further back, just to be 'on the safe side', but all memories from before that sack race were relatively benign. When his mother's extrovert way of being became apparent, every so often, it merely produced a grin. There was no sign of any foot waggling, and he could talk about the sack race (and any of the other recalls) with no discomfort. In all, he had had four sessions, plus an initial consultation, and pronounced himself 'well pleased!'

It is not necessary to enlarge here upon the links between each substituted symptom, because you should be able to discover them for yourself if you are not already aware of them—by reading through the case again. It is obvious that he began his symptoms when he was under pressure and failed, and suffered the start of his current symptom some 25 years later when circumstances echoed that originating event. Most symptom substitution will occur when something new is being undertaken.

Not every client, of course, will be as obliging and easy to work with as this one was, and it may be necessary to hunt about quite a bit before you find the clue to carry you back to the next symptom. Where your client presents with more than one symptom, it may be necessary to work through each of them in the same way; when this is the case, though, you will often find the answer in just one session. Always adopt the same mode of behaviour:

(1) Search for the first occurrences of the current symptom.

(2) Give the symptom permission and reason to exist.

(3) Establish what 'it' was doing before the current symptom—in other words, find out what the previous symptom was.

(4) Explore/find this previous symptom by examining what was happening in your client's life at that time

(5) Seek the first occurrence of this symptom. If this seems not to be the originating event, then go back to step (2).

Originating anxiety

The easiest way for you to be certain that you have released the originating anxiety is that your client should be able to talk about *any* of the events he has recalled with no discomfort or emotion, or any physical signs via body language that all is not well.

Perhaps the most important thing to remember with this technique is to consider the symptom as being a separate entity and always refer to it as such with your client. He will soon become accustomed to this and will begin to subconsciously accept that *he is not his symptom*. Once there is the recognition of the existence of substituted symptomatic processes, the analytical, logically-minded client will become engrossed in the search and will *truly want* to find out what was happening before his current problems showed themselves. It is not at all unusual, in fact, for the client to arrive for his session already aware of the next stage back, having had it 'pop into his mind' during the time since he last saw you. In this case, you could start with step (4), above.

There are many ways you can guide the conversation with your client, and you will need to be alert to catch every opportunity to 'home in' on the originating event, always seeking to place the emotion/response there because it *wanted* to be there or had just cause to be there. The 'conversational' interludes work best when they *sound* like normal conversation, since this will help to get the client's subconscious off-guard. You should be careful, though, to keep rigorously to what the client has told you and use his own language patterns, e.g.: client calls stomach 'gut' so therapist calls stomach 'gut'; client calls stomach 'tummy' so therapist calls stomach 'tummy'.

Finally, it is very important to ensure that, as with any other form of regression/analytical therapy, you use only the cleanest of language in your communications with your client (see Chapter 10).

Chapter 23

Ancestral Archetypes and Modelling

While it is not investigative or analytical by nature, the work shown in this chapter can produce a startlingly rapid and permanent change for many people. It is based upon the ability of the mind to 'anchor' resources but, unlike some other forms of this type of work, we are going to allow the client to discover for herself that the resources she needs *already exist* within her psyche.

It is particularly well-suited to the client who perceives her problem as annoying, rather than properly distressing. Most forms of social phobia, difficulties with personal interaction, problems with assertiveness or decision making, the inability to say 'no', and situation-specific fears are all good examples, though the technique has also been effective with other, more serious, conditions. Since it uses a conscious link to the subconscious, it is not recommended where there is an autonomic response such as panic syndrome, sweating palms, spontaneous vomiting, IBS (Irritable Bowel Syndrome), migraine headaches and the like.

*It should **not** be used to assist a client to override clinical symptoms, especially those where pain is associated.*

The technique is based around the concept of ancestral memory, inherited potential for behaviour, and skills that your client may have no awareness of at the time when she presents for treatment. A bit of scene-setting is necessary at the beginning, and the easiest way to do this is to outline the way that our particular species evolved from its earliest beginnings, around one hundred thousand years ago. Some guidance is given here.

Before the beginning

Although we know that hominids first appeared on earth around three million years or more ago, there is no proof that those creatures were actually our direct ancestors. Some scientists believe we are related to the very early species and/or to the later

185

Neanderthal and Cro-Magnon man, while others believe that we are a separate race entirely, first appearing between ninety thousand and no earlier than two hundred thousand years ago. It does not much matter, really, as far as we are concerned. If we are related, then we have inherited their savagery; if we are not, then we had enough of our own to deal with theirs, for they were around until about thirty thousand years ago, by which time Modern Man appears to have become an established species.

Since those earliest days of *Homo sapiens sapiens*, there have been hundreds of generations of violence, plagues, famine, witches, warlocks and wizards, crusades, wars, fantastic inventions and even more fantastic events. Interbreeding has passed on mixed genetics; environment has ensured a goodly amount of neurosis and general anxiety. So truly, each and every human being is unique, because the computations of the effects of the environment upon the genetic exchanges are almost infinite. And when you take a look at the whole evolutionary process on a percentage basis, it is no wonder that we, all of us, still exhibit primitive behaviour quite often.

The wandering savage

Homo sapiens sapiens was nomadic in existence, living in groups of twenty-five to fifty individuals, until about ten thousand years ago, when some, the **Settlers**, began to learn how to farm and domesticate plants and animals. These were the earliest attempts at civilisation. This was a gift for the less developed, more brutal individuals who had always lived by the rule of kill or be killed, for they could simply take over and control each settlement. They soon became the **Warriors** of this new era. There were others who had no stomach for fighting and whose restlessness militated against the slow business of agricultural development; they reverted to the behaviour patterns of their earliest ancestors and opted for an unencumbered life of roaming the world, becoming the **Nomads.**

These three 'tribes' the Warriors, the Settlers and the Nomads are still very much with us today and although they present themselves in a modern form, with modern behaviour patterns, they are not so very much different in nature from those early ancestors. We all possess something of each of them and you will shortly learn of the enormous importance of this recognition.

Once civilisation had started, everything proceeded apace with much interbreeding of these three main 'tribes'. We know little of the daily reality of these people, since the first written language appeared only in 3500 BC, developed by the Sumerians and the Ancient Egyptians. Everything prior to that is considered to be pre-historic and it is hard to know exactly how the human race behaved. What is certain, though, is that even being generous and assuming that our particular race did not appear until around one hundred thousand years ago, we are still no more than ten per cent 'modern'. Ninety per cent of our psycho-genetic make-up has not even reached the level of the barbarous middle-ages and by far the vast majority of it is still that of a wandering savage. Evolution moves slowly and it will be a long time yet before the human animal truly becomes as we try already to be.

In the meantime, most humans are going to be born with conflict—or potential for conflict—already in place, the resolution of which is unlikely to occur at birth but probably as and when needed, or maybe even never. Perhaps, in the rare situation where there is no conflict, either within or externally, this may result in the superconfident personality, the 'together' person who finds the process of living an easy one to cope with from the very beginning and who tends to be successful in most of her undertakings. The one who makes living look easy, in fact, simply because it *is* easy, since her ancestral urges are in harmony with her existence, allowing the individual to easily adapt, control, or simply not care.

This ancestral memory concept is well-established in nature; it is known that the offspring of rats who have been taught to find their way through a maze learn to find *their* way through that same maze more quickly than their parents did. And *their* progeny find it easier still. Eels know how to get to the Sargasso sea to breed, though they have never been there before. Birds know migration routes. Nature abounds with examples of the existence of ancestral memory, not the least of which is the established fact that twins who are separated at birth will often have astonishingly similar lives and lifestyles as they grow up. The way they tackle life and the process of living may have been moulded by parent figures, but the way they *feel*, the things they like and their reactions to adversity will often be astoundingly similar.

The modern versions

Now, the modern versions of those three tribes usually behave somewhat differently from their ancient counterparts *but the instincts for that behaviour are still present in the psyche.* A full breakdown of each type is given in Chapter Three, on personality, in which you will see that there are descriptive 'professional' names for each. The Warrior is the **Resolute Organisational** personality (RO for short); the Settler has the title of **Intuitive Adaptable** (IA), while the Nomad is **Charismatic Evidential** (CE). For this chapter, though, we will keep to the 'user-friendly' names of Warrior, Settler and Nomad. In the 'thumbnail' descriptions which follow, the negative attributes of each type are ignored, since we need the positive aspects to help our clients.

The **Modern Warrior** is ambitious and goal-directed, can be somewhat selfish and seeks to be in control of self and everybody else. Warriors have a firm, no-nonsense attitude to life and living and are able to stand their ground quite easily. Because they are not overly concerned with pleasing others, there is no problem with stating their case or saying 'no' when necessary. There are often good organisational skills linked to great practicality. The Warrior likes things she can see, touch and understand.

The **Modern Settler** is a 'people person' who is not overly ambitious and just wants to be comfortable and secure. Communicative, extraordinarily adaptable and easy-going, settlers are the 'nice' people of the world, responsive and caring, and among the most sociable of souls. They seek the best in people and often find it, as well as having a happy knack of making friends easily and finding solutions to all sorts of personal difficulties with ease. There is often a quick grasp of how to avoid the recurrence of awkward situations.

The **Modern Nomad** often seems larger than life and, indeed, likes to be 'in the limelight', quite easily being the life and soul of the party. Nomads' somewhat extrovert manner means that they have little or no difficulty as far as interaction with others is concerned and they can make excellent public speakers, actors, illusionists and the like. They are particularly good at anything which requires a dramatic or 'up front' approach and are usually uninhibitedly spontaneous.

Every generation carries genetic information from each of the three main character types, but there is usually one set of genes that is dominant, shaping our personality, the way we conduct our life, the partners that we choose, our careers, and so on. Or, rather, the way we *should* conduct our life, our careers, the partners we *should* choose. Because here is the great difficulty, possibly one of the main reasons for neurosis: *genetic selection is a random process, so progeny may very well not be from the same 'tribe' as their parents.* Warriors, for instance, can produce Settlers or Nomads. And those parents will attempt to rear the child with *their* values, diluting and distorting the inborn instincts and resources. The child then has the choice of believing implicitly what she is taught or told, suppressing all natural instincts to the contrary *and suffering neurosis as a result*; or following her natural instincts in spite of the admonishment of parents and others, doing what feels right and seems natural, only to eventually end up with the enforced belief that she is a 'rebel' or somehow 'not right', maybe unlovable... *and suffering neurosis as a result*.

Yet the sad thing is, all the resources for success are there in the psyche, inherited from the times when just to survive was, in itself, success. If we can find a way to tap into those resources, we can help our clients find something of their true selves.

Application

It is actually entirely possible to learn how to access the ancestral instincts of each of those three tribes as and when necessary, allowing us to be effective over a far wider range of activities and situations than we might otherwise manage.

Having outlined the concept of inherited ancestral memories, ask your client which of the three types she believes would be best equipped to deal with whatever situation it is that has brought her to you. You might need to help her decide, so memorise a few of the following examples.

Warriors: Celtic Kings and Chieftains, Warrior Queens, Normans, Vikings, Crusaders, Knights, Native Indians, Samurai, Zulus, Shoguns, Trojans, Nubian Kings and Queens, Roman Gladiators and Centurions, Chinese and Japanese Emperors, Ancient Huns, Saxons, Gurkhas.

Settlers: Homesteaders, Ancient Farmers, Livestock Workers, Ancient Builders, Carers of all descriptions, Healers, Craftsmen of all types, Teachers, Monks, Nuns, Prophets and Seers, Clothiers and Dressmakers, Barbers, Shopkeepers, Researchers, Philosophers, Artists, Musicians, Composers and 'Searchers for Truth'.

Nomads: Gypsies, Wandering Minstrels, Tinkers, Ancient Arabs, Actors, Tricksters, Travellers, Sorcerers, Witches, Warlocks, Wizards, Itinerant Musicians, Soothsayers, fake Prophets and Seers, minor Thieves and Pick-pockets, Pirates, Highwaymen, Outlaws, Court Jesters, Story-tellers, Dancers, Magicians and Conjurors, Illusionists.

When the client has chosen, help her to develop an image of such a character, seeking an early archetype which may be a fictional hero, a character from history, or simply an invention of her own imagination. Ideally, we need an 'ancient' character, rather than a modern one; this is not a role-playing exercise. Using hypnosis, help your client to develop a Vivid Mental Image (VMI) to the point where she can begin to feel as if she must have known this person. It is not unusual for a client to eventually observe: "I think I must have based this on someone I know…"

Vivid imagery

This image must be as vivid as possible; the way the character looks, sounds, moves, acts etc. For instance, a client imagining a Warrior might visualise an inscrutable oriental with a colourful costume and mystic skills; or a foot soldier of the Roman legions; or perhaps a stealthy hunter who is neither seen nor heard until it is too late. The Settler might be based more on 'feel'—perhaps a character who is in touch with her emotions and not ashamed of them. Settler men can be gentle and kind. Settler women can be angry. Either can rage against any form of injustice and either can forgive transgressions and let bygones be bygones. Nomads... well, the great thing about the archetypal Nomad is the sense of fun and spontaneity, and the ability to project her personality well. When the modern Nomad possesses this ability, that is the individual with real charisma.

Use your and your client's imagination to the full, and use your own personality to make the exercise *fun.*

Once the image has been created and developed, it is important that you point out that anything you can imagine is based upon a reality somewhere in your mind, even if you are not consciously aware of that reality. Anything your mind produces is a product of how your mind works. And since the client has created this archetypal personality from the ancestral memories present in her own mind, she must therefore have available to her the resources that that character would have possessed, the resources which she herself believes would help her to overcome her difficulties. Identify how that resource would be used when she needs it and use visualisation techniques to reinforce the belief.

Now comes the truly important bit! While the client is still in hypnosis, repeat several times the suggestion that it is only necessary for her to create the VMI of that archetype and hold it in her mind for a few seconds, *and she will instantly have available to her all the resources of that archetype.*

Here are two case studies that illustrate the technique.

Case study 1

Dave was in his late thirties, involved in the arms industry, and quite often required to make major presentations of computer software that had been developed by his team. The problem was, that while he was an expert when it came to organising and developing the necessary work to a completed level, when it came to the presentation part, he had a big problem.

He blushed furiously as soon as he stood up to speak.

This was not a slight pink glow, but a ferocious scarlet that was accompanied by sweating, voice tremors, and waves of nausea that would start when it became apparent that those present could observe his discomfort. It would carry on until he reached the closing moments of his dissertation, when it would abruptly subside to leave him feeling perfectly in control. In all other areas of his life he claimed to be confident and at ease. He presented himself for therapy just one week before his next 'performance'.

He was immediately fascinated by the idea of ancestral memories and the concept of the Warrior, Settler and Nomad tribes and identified himself accurately as a Settler/Warrior combination, with 'hardly any Nomad at all'. He recognised that it was this absence of Nomad personality traits which was making it difficult for him to be 'up front', because he did not much like anything which required him to project himself in any way. He did not see himself as an inspiring personality at all.

We discussed the options: using the Settler self to develop confidence in the communicative skills, or the Warrior self for the ability to stand his ground. He decided that the idea of using the Warrior felt better and so we decided to go with that.

It took him no longer than thirty seconds to decide that his archetypal Warrior was Genghis Khan; this is a common choice, though the actual image varies enormously from one individual to another. In hypnosis, Dave easily described a VMI of 'his' Genghis Khan: oriental and somewhat like a Samurai but even tougher, with metallic-looking garb, dark skin, and carrying an inscrutable expression about him. His sword was sheathed and he was confident enough that he only really needed to draw it in battle; the rest of the time, he would simply survey his situation with the calmness that comes from knowing that you are invincible. When necessary, he could clearly describe his plans with the precision of a general in command of an army. A truly formidable individual!

When asked, in hypnosis, how likely Genghis Khan would be to blush when he presented his ideas to an assembly, Dave burst out laughing and said that it simply could not happen. Quite apart from the dark skin, he would know his plans were good and beyond doubt. "Anyway," he added, "He would *know* that it was him who was in control."

He agreed that he actually felt quite empowered by the image that he had created and enjoyed the thought, given as a suggestion, that he would only have to visualise this character to be able to access the positive resources that he needed, whilst still acting very much as his *'real self, the confident self, the self that knows just what to do and just how to do it…'* etc. The suggestion was repeated several times, interspersed with imagery of him presenting his talk with total calmness, the knowledge that he was in control and that his plans had been made well and were totally effective. This 'echoing' of the qualities attributed to the archetype by the client is a very powerful method of maximising the effect of suggestion.

Two days after his presentation, he telephoned to say that he had actually *enjoyed* the experience for the first time ever and was looking forward to the next one!

Case study 2

Susan used the process almost by accident! Forty-six years old, estranged from her husband and temporarily living with her mother, she had presented with a problem with concentration and memory—she was studying for a new career in photography at her local college and was having trouble in retaining the information, even though she easily understood it. In addition to her presenting problem, she also tended towards mild insomnia and occasional bouts of nausea. All the symptoms had only shown up relatively recently; before that, she had had no particular problems since her late twenties, when she had suffered some IBS problems and panic attacks. Between then and now she had lived abroad, and although her symptoms only started when she returned to this country, she did not believe that this was relevant.

We decided that hypnoanalysis was the way to resolve her problems and began with a standard presentation of the concept of ancestral memory, and Warriors, Settlers and Nomads, etc. When asked what she believed she might be, she replied almost instantly that she was a Settler but then added that she thought she was a 'closet Nomad.' This was interesting, because the symptom pattern suggested the CE, or Nomad personality type, as did much of her demeanour. But she had always been punished as a child, she said, for any form of extrovert behaviour, both parents insisting that any form of 'showing off' was totally undesirable. Words, smacks and manipulation (maternal affection being totally withheld for any breaches of the required behaviour) had eventually led to her always behaving 'like a nice girl should'. At this point, she became embarrassed and said that she had actually been a bit of a tomboy in her early years and she thought that her mother did not consider her feminine enough.

With one of those moments of insight that we all know and love, the therapist asked if Mum considered photography to be a feminine pursuit; Susan flustered and asked if that meant she were a lesbian!

The next week saw a totally different woman enter the consulting room; the rather staid frock that she had worn the week before had been replaced by leather trousers and a fluorescent orange blouse; she wore a colourful chiffon scarf around her neck, huge gold hoop earrings, and her hair was darker and piled up on top of her head—and she looked great! A truly Charismatic Evidential character!

"What d'you think?" she said, posing in the middle of the consulting room. "It's my new image. Don't you think I look really arty?"

"It suits you. What happened?"

"Ah, well, it was you talking about all those Warriors and Nomads," she replied. "When I left here, I got thinking I must've been a gypsy dancer in a past life or something. I could see her as clearly as anything. She was a bit... well... *wild*, really." She fingered her earrings as she spoke, and looked a bit thoughtful. "And do you know," she continued, "it's a really strange thing, but I was quite suddenly completely unconcerned about whatever my stuffy old mother thinks about what I do with my life—and I didn't even know I'd *been* concerned!"

Without knowing it, Susan had anchored into one of the resources associated with the Nomad: a light-hearted rejection of anything that was stuffy, staid, or conformist. We actually completed a successful analysis after that, but the moment she created the archetype of the Gypsy dancer was the moment at which she began to get free of those childhood restrictions. At the last session she was waxing enthusiastic about her progress in the photography class and promised to send some examples of her work—which she never did. Typical CE trait!

While this application of the ancestral memory concept should not replace analysis or regression, these two case histories illustrate (a) how it can be used as a 'quick fix' for a single problem that may have more to do with situations than psychological damage; and (b) how it can be used to give a 'kick start' to analytical therapy. This tends to be a spontaneous event, though it can easily be engineered by any therapist with a bit of imagination.

Chapter 24

Three Useful Short Routines

The three routines here can be very helpful in speeding the course of therapy. The rapid cognitive interrupt routine makes for easy desensitising of a stimulus; the bonding routine makes for increased transference phenomena, as does the 'I believe' script.

Rapid cognitive interrupt

There are times when a client will say to you: "I just can't seem to stop seeing his face… it's always there in my mind." Sometimes it might be a particular scene that 'keeps coming back', or maybe a sound. The pattern interrupt method employed here to help alleviate such problems is quick, effective and versatile enough that it may even be used to help successfully manage some of the symptoms of PTSD (Post Traumatic Stress Disorder). As you will see, it is a true 'hands-on' therapeutic procedure.

We will assume, for the purpose of this description of the technique, that your client is 'stuck' with the image of somebody's face for some reason—this is actually not uncommon in some cases of emotional abuse. On occasions, the face may appear in the individual's mind only when trying to perform a particular task or behaviour: buying a personal item, meeting new people, going into unfamiliar places, sexual activity—all are common situations where this might occur. It is quite possible that your client had not realised that he was suffering this particular problem until it had been revealed by other therapeutic methods.

To begin, have your client seated facing you (a straight-backed chair works best), arms extended towards you, palms upwards with fingers together, eyes open and raised to look towards the ceiling. You will stand immediately in front of him, close enough so that you can easily reach his fingertips. Now proceed:

Therapist: Okay, now I want you to think of that face. Keep looking up at the ceiling, and imagine you can see that face up there, as vividly as you can. Can you see that face now?

Wait until your client confirms this.

Therapist: Good. Okay, now just keep focused on that face for as long as you can...

Now you reach out and *rapidly* 'bat' your client's hands with yours. Use a fairly firm action and a rhythm of around four to six actions per second; only your fingers should contact your client's hand/fingers, not your palms.

Therapist: Keep looking at that face. What's happening to it?

Client: It's breaking up.

Therapist: (continuing the action) *That's right. It's breaking up... tell me what's happening now.*

It should not be long before your client tells you that the face 'has gone'. Of course, you will keep up the physical action until this happens—and it *will* happen, because it is almost impossible to feel two active stimuli without one seeking to become part of, or associated with, the other. The rapid stop-start stimulus of the hands will cause a similar effect to occur in the imagery centres of the brain and the visual image will fractionate, then dissolve. It may, of course, return later on but it will be less dominant and will respond more quickly the second time. After a third 'treatment' (and this will not always be necessary) it will simply cease to occur.

Bonding (between therapist and client)

This useful routine is adapted from a technique used by the famous American hypnotherapist, Milton H. Erickson. It can dramatically increase transference, especially when used at or near the beginning of therapy.

Begin with your favourite induction, then continue:

"Stay deeply relaxed and enjoy these feelings of calmness and peace and allow your whole being to go still deeper down to enjoy the level of relaxation that your body needs and enjoys feeling.

*"Your mind may wander off occasionally but there's no reason to let that bother you... This is a process for complete and total relaxation and calmness in the body **and** in the mind, and because of this, that wonderful hypnotic feeling will still continue to increase.*

*"Your mind can hear, and is hearing, the sound of my voice on two levels...on a conscious everyday level and on a **deeper subconscious level**, so that if your mind wanders off, that's okay. Don't let that bother you.*

*"My voice will travel along with you, and it doesn't matter where you go my voice will go along with you, my voice will flow and travel along with you, my voice can even assume the identity of someone else, someone you know, or **someone you will imagine**... Always someone you can deeply relate to... Always someone you can show all your emotions to... Always someone you can express those emotions to...*

(pause)

"And that's okay.

"That's right.

*"So that **you will**, always, continue to respond to me on a subconscious level, no **matter where you are**.*

"Relax and be still now while your powerful subconscious mind links and connects with the sound of my voice.

(pause)

*"Your subconscious mind knows what it has to do... so, you see, there is nothing whatsoever for you to do consciously... the process will happen **automatically**, just as certainly as your next outbreath.*

"That's right.

"Relax now, and go still deeper with every word I speak."

Now continue with the session just as you would normally.

The 'I believe' script

This ego-strengthener is based around work by E.A. Barnett, MD. The constant requests for confirmation encourage transference, self-belief and belief in the therapist, and the subject-matter encourages self-realisation and an increased sense of self-worth. The willingness of the therapist to accept any differences also encourages transference. It is useful, though not essential, to set up an ideomotor response for this script before you begin.

After a suitable induction and deepener, continue with:

"I believe that every human being is unique and important. **Do you agree?**"

Here, the client has the choice to either confirm or deny that he agrees with this statement. If there is disagreement, we need to change the thought processes slightly to remove that sense of disagreement. Once this has been done, resistance is dramatically lowered. This is actually quite easy to do and the same method could be used almost anywhere within the technique. In this case, we would proceed with:

"Even though you disagree with me..."

before continuing with:

"Do you believe me when I say... **I** believe every human being to be important and unique?"

Disagreement here reveals the form of resistance where the client is *determined* the therapist's efforts are to be in vain. To help deal with this, study Chapter 7, which includes advice on releasing resistance. This difficulty will need to be resolved before you can make any true progress with this client. Assuming all is well, however, continue with:

"I believe that you (client's name) *are unique and special—just as unique and important as any other human being living or dead.* **Do you agree?"**

Here, the client will be pretty much compelled to agree, if only for the reason that the therapist has, only a few seconds previously, obtained his acceptance of the therapist's belief structure. This is where we can usefully employ the ideomotor response, if we have not already been doing so. Continue:

"Is there any part of your entire mind that does not agree with me?"

Disagreement being shown will need to be worked through in some way before continuing with the following clinchers for improved self-worth and acceptance:

"I believe that you (client's name) *have the right to* **all** *of your feelings whether or not they are unpleasant.* **Do you agree?"**

Wait for confirmation—as long as it takes.

"I believe that you have as much right to your feelings of sadness as any other human being, as much right to your feelings of happiness as any other human being, as much right to your feelings of anger as any other human being, as much right to your love, your fear and your safe feelings. **Do you agree?"**

Wait for confirmation.

"I believe that you do not need to feel guilty, ashamed or embarrassed about any of your normal human emotions… you have the absolute right to keep them for as long as you need them and the absolute right to let them go when they are no longer necessary. **Do you agree?"**

Having now confirmed that he is at least the equal of any other person and that his emotional states are valid and acceptable, the client will be far more responsive to whatever change-work is required.

Chapter 25

Four Useful End-of-Therapy Routines

The old repeats

The main objective of this technique is to enable your client to go over all the work you have completed and trace anything which may be remaining and which needs to be worked through, or anything which may have been missed during the sessions. You would use this technique in the last session to assess the completion of therapy.

This technique can also be used to enable your client to see the effect that a childhood experience has had on her adult life. In this case you would ask her to put the originating image on to the screen, then allow her unconscious mind to take over and project on to the screen all the different ways in which it has tried to show her—perhaps the people who have been drawn into her life or the places and circumstances she has found herself in. Use an appropriate induction taking your client to a room and then proceed as follows:

> *"As you step inside this room your comfort-level doubles and you feel safe. Be sure to close the door behind you, no one else may enter this place, just you and the sound of my voice. The lighting here is soft and soothing just take a moment and notice its colour—perhaps it is a yellow or a powdery blue. I don't know what colour it is but you do.*
>
> *"In front of you, you can see a large and very relaxing chair. Make your way slowly and lazily towards the chair and feel yourself becoming calmer and calmer as you get closer and closer.*
>
> *"Now make yourself really comfortable in the chair and as you make yourself really comfortable, look ahead of you. You can see a screen, a large screen, sort of like an old cinema screen and in the top left-hand corner is a dull-looking, red light.*

"You will notice that the screen is blank at the moment and that it has a shiny sheen to it - similar to the colour of the light. Focus now on your right hand resting on the arm of the chair. In your right hand you are holding the controls, just like video controls, you know, a little hand set of push buttons like FAST FORWARD, REWIND, PAUSE, STOP and START.

"Now focus on your left hand because you are going to see something that you haven't noticed before. Right there, by your hand, is a beautiful glove. It's made of the finest silk fabric and I want you to just let your left hand slowly slip into the glove, that's right. Notice how well it fits you, how comfortable it is. And I want you to notice something else about this glove, too, something very important because there is a loose thread, a fine and delicate thread, and that thread is connected to the screen. And in a moment I shall tell you why. In just a little while you are going to review on the screen every negative moment which has occurred during the time we have spent together. Every memory that you have recalled of every incident which has given you a negative feeling or behaviour or reaction.

"If something should appear on the screen which you have not seen before, the red light will start to flash very brightly and you will need to tell me what it is that you are seeing.

"If anything appears on the screen which gives you an uncomfortable feeling or a feeling of discomfort in anyway, then you will experience that emotion directly through the glove via the loose thread attached to the screen. And you will need to tell me what it is you are feeling.

"In a moment I shall ask you to push the START button. You will be able to review everything surprisingly quickly. I shall remain here in silence.

"When the red light flashes or when you experience any emotion through the glove just let me know. Do you understand? "

Pause and wait for client's response.

"Thank you. All right, push the START button now and let me know when the process is complete by just nodding your head."

You should always have the glove on the left hand because this is the 'feeling' side of the body. It makes little difference if your client is left-handed or right-handed. Give your client the time she needs and observe her carefully for signs of discomfort, because if she did not tell you something the first time round, she may decide to not tell you this time either!

The stepping-into-life technique

This script may be used to evaluate the client's progress at the end of therapy. Use an appropriate induction and then proceed as follows:

"Now I want you to imagine yourself standing at the entrance to a long, dark corridor. And look down that corridor towards a small circle of bright light at the far end. Imagine yourself, as vividly as you can, moving forward into that corridor - moving forward along that corridor towards that circle of bright light at the far end. Just imagine that circle of bright light just moving closer and getting larger and brighter. Moving closer, getting larger and brighter. Until that circle of bright light is so close, so large, so bright that you are just one step away from it. One step away from stepping into that circle of bright light.

"And in this light allow yourself to notice a door. At first the light comes from under the door. And then you notice the light outlining the door. And then you, perhaps, notice that there is something written on the door. A word—the word LIFE—written in large gold or silvery letters on the door, there for you to read. That word LIFE inviting you towards the door. Are you ready to receive life, to pass through that door and to accept everything that life has to offer in the present? Not past illusions or future dreams but life in the present in all its challenging but endlessly-fascinating reality.

"Maybe at first you could feel a part of you which may be scared to accept this invitation or, perhaps, there is a small part of you which feels unworthy and thus unable to accept it. But maybe this will only be a passing thought. Take this opportunity now. Embrace it, welcome it, rejoice in it and step through that door."

Here is some guidance for one or two possibilities that may arise:

> **Therapist:** *Tell me, can you step out through that door at the end of the corridor?*
>
> **Client:**
>
> **Therapist:** *Tell me, tell me truthfully, can you step out through that door at the end of this corridor?*
>
> **Client:** Yes.
>
> **Therapist:** *Tell me what you can see and tell me what you feel.*

Continue as appropriate.

> Or:
>
> **Client:** No.
>
> **Therapist:** *Do you see anything or do you feel anything?*
>
> **Client:** Yes.
>
> **Therapist:** *Tell me what you see and tell me what you feel.*

Continue as appropriate.

> Or:
>
> **Client:** No.
>
> **Therapist:** *That's fine, don't worry. I want you to let your mind drift and wander, wander and drift anywhere it wants to.*

In this way, your client will be able to start free-association again and continue with the analysis. Sometimes a client may claim that she cannot step out through the door because she is frightened or for some other reason she is unable to do so. Whatever the client says, use this as a starting point to continue the analysis.

The race-for-life technique

The following script is most suitable for use at the end of therapy. It is very moving, motivating and uplifting for your client and is a wonderful way to conclude your sessions. As the race begins, you are the commentator; keep the pace fast, the tempo up and be there.

Relax your client and proceed as follows:

> *"And I want you to focus and notice a warm and welcoming darkness. That's right, a warm and welcoming darkness on the inside of your mind. You feel safe and free here. And as you imagine yourself in this warm and welcoming darkness, you notice in front of you now far, far in the distance a tiny pinprick of white light. Far in the distance just a tiny pinprick of white light. And as you focus and notice this tiny pinprick of white light, you begin to hear the gentle sound of whispering voices. Just a few at first and as you notice a few you begin to hear more and more.*
>
> *"You look around now and see people, lots and lots of people and they are all different. Some are tall and some short, some thin, some fat, some light, some dark, male, female, blond hair, red hair, brown hair. All different. And you notice the feeling of excitement and anticipation in the air. It's as if you can just breathe it in and your breathing is calm, even and relaxed. Focus again on the light far in the distance, just look at the pinprick of light and sense its magnetism. It's as if it's drawing you towards it even though you are not moving yet.*
>
> *"You notice the people next to you stretching and warming up as if they are going to run. They are wearing sports clothes, shorts and vests, that sort of thing. All bright colours. You look at yourself and notice what you are wearing as you also begin to prepare to run towards the light. Prepare to run the race of your life. You're going to run like you've never run before. You're going to run the race of your life against 50,000 other people to the light.*
>
> *"Get ready and on the count of 3 you run.*
>
> *"One, two, three—**Go!***

"Go on—run. Faster, faster, faster. That's right, go on faster and faster and faster. You've got to win. Faster and faster and faster. You feel good. Your body is strong. Feel the power in your legs pounding with every stride you make as if you are a gazelle. Use your arms, move your body. Come on, faster and faster, that's right. Keep going faster and faster and faster. Someone's fallen over, jump over that person, jump over that person, that's right, keep going, keep going. They're falling down all over the place, keep going. They can't take the pace, keep going.

"There are 40,000 and you, 40,000 and you. And you know you can do it. You feel the wind behind you and the magnetism of the light drawing you closer. And look at the light, as you get closer, it gets bigger and bigger. You feel its energy, its awesome power. Someone's grabbed your arm, pull away from that person, pull away and go faster. There's a gap there on the outside - go for it, get in that space, go on, go for it, go for it. That's right, faster and faster.

"There are 30,000 and you, 30,000 and you. You feel good—you've paced yourself. Lungs are powerful, legs strong, adrenaline pumping through your body now. Every muscle doing what it should. Every fibre and tissue of your very being healthy and alive. Keep going, that's right. Faster and faster. Someone has fallen over, oh, and they're all piling into each other, go round them, go round them. Nothing can stand in your way, go round them. Good.

"There are 20,000 and you, 20,000 and you. Closer and closer towards the light—its magnetism—just drawing you closer and closer. It radiates out to you as if it's calling to you. All your senses are alive and vibrant. Run faster and faster. You feel good. You know you can do it! Go on, run! Run!

"Someone's left some old rubbish in your path, look, up ahead—some rubble and cans and rotten stuff you can't even recognise anymore. Jump it, you're ready, jump over it, jump. Yes. Leave it far behind now. Look to the light and run. Faster and faster. Faster and faster. GO. GO. GO. GO. Run. Come on, run! Faster!

"10,000 and you, 10,000 and you. Look at the light, feel it drawing you closer and, at the same time, you can experience all the sensations in your body. Your determination—you know it's always been there. The ease of the power in your limbs, natural. Your heart strong and enjoying life. Your mind focused on your path… Run, come on now, run! There are 5,000 and you. Come on, let's go, go, go! Feel that freedom inside you and know that you can express it with your body. Just let go and run. Faster and faster. That's right. Faster, faster, faster.

"There are 2,000 and you, just 2,000 and you. You're still feeling strong, it's getting easier and easier for you. Look at the others sitting on the side, just look at them, they can't keep up, they weren't ready, they're falling down all over the place. Faster and faster. Faster and faster.

"There are 500 now and you. You can see the front. You're almost there. Faster and faster. Come on, get up the front, get up the front. Run, run, run. Faster now faster.

"Oh, and look at the light. It's huge. You're almost there. Look at it radiating out—endless and serene. Silent and powerful all at the same time.

"One hundred and you. The light drawing you closer. Faster and faster. Hear your feet pounding with every stride, you can hear your own breathing, you're centred and focused. You can do it, you are doing it. That's right. Faster and faster. Faster and faster. Nothing and no one's gonna stop you now!

"Fifty others and you. Faster, faster, faster. Run now, run. Get up the front. Get to the front. Come on. The others are breathless but you can do it. You've paced yourself, you feel good. Go on faster and faster and faster. Nothing's gonna stop you now.

"Forty, 30, 20, 10 others and you. They're falling down all over the place. Jump over, go round, find that space, get through there whatever it takes get there. Go on, faster and faster. Run like the wind. It's as if your feet aren't touching the ground any more. Look at the light, it's all around you now.

"Run, run, run, run. You're almost there, go on faster, faster, run! RUN! Two. One. Get in front, get to the front, that's right. Yes, take *the lead. Go on, go, go, go. That's right. Nothing and no one in front of you now. Just the light.*

"Prepare to jump into the light. Prepare to jump into the light. Get ready, you're there, that's right. And jump, jump into the light. You've won. You've won! Against 50,000 others you won."

Now change pace to a soothing one and continue:

"Rest now, float and relax in the light. The light supporting you as if by some magical, unseen energy. Here is where you rest and heal and revitalise yourself as you prepare to claim your prize. Within the light you breathe in love, harmony, strength, wisdom, understanding, joy. For the light is the experience of everything you need. Breathe gently now and allow your body to rest and absorb all that you need.

"Imagine you've been in the light for one week. Your body continues to heal and revitalise itself. You experience now the sensation of just letting it happen naturally, the way nature intended it to be..."

(short pause)

"Now you have been in the light for one month. There is a calmness within you which you have perhaps never experienced before and, at the same time, it's as if an awakening is occurring. Just drift and float and let it happen naturally for you. That's right."

(short pause)

"You have been drifting in the light for three months now. Your body healing and revitalising, forming and developing. Every muscle, fibre and tissue of your body, every organ and every bone, every artery and every vein healthy and functioning just as it should for you. Blood flows easily, cleansing processes occur automatically. And you just relax."

(short pause)

"You have been in the light for four months and you are mentally and physically stronger than you have ever before experienced.

Breathe in all that you need: insight, love, success, power, under-standing, patience, joy, happiness, wisdom. It's all there for you to absorb. And that feeling that you know you need, that feeling that only you know you need, breathe it in now. Focus and notice now how your skin also absorbs. Notice also the suppleness and elasticity of your skin and how clear and fresh your skin is."

(short pause)

"You have been gently drifting in the light for six months now. Your natural and instinctive senses of touch, smell, vision, taste and hearing are all so clear and so fresh. And you feel that sixth sense naturally beginning to open up like a beautiful flower-bud. Your whole being beginning to blossom and flower. It's like the most beautiful garden you have ever seen, where water flows gently on its journey. The sun shines every day. Flowers of the brightest, vibrant colours and fragrances. Somewhere in the distance you can hear the gentle tinkling sound of chimes dancing in a warm breeze. The most beautiful place, right there in your very being."

(short pause)

"You have been in the light now for eight months. Your mind and body feel ready to claim your prize. Focus and notice yourself with your limbs strong, healthy and perfectly formed—every organ of your being revitalised and fresh. Your skin supple, clean and clear. Your breathing easy and effortless. Eyes bright, radiating with the life within you.

"Breathe in the light, breathe in all that you need, for soon it will be time to leave this place and move forward. Breathe in life. Breathe in love and joy, peace and hope. Breathe in strength and determination. Breathe in wisdom and enlightenment. Breathe in achievement and success. Breathe in delight and rapture. Breathe in fulfilment and pleasure. Breathe it all in—absorb from the light what you need."

Pause for approximately 10 seconds.

"Now you have been in the light for nine months and it is time to leave this place. And as you leave this place you may experience a rushing sensation. It will be a momentary experience for you to

> *enjoy. You now have everything that you need to move forward. Feel the rush and step into a beautiful place of nature. Feel grass beneath your feet and warm sunshine on your skin. Stand tall and be at one with nature. Look around you at the natural beauty."*

Pause for approximately 3 seconds.

> *"For this is your prize—the gift of life. Against 50,000 others you won. That's right, you won. You are a winner. A winner of life. Claim your prize now, hold it in your hands and in your heart, free to live your life your way, for there is no other way to live your life but your way. You are a winner of life, to be a winner in life."*

Now conclude the session.

This last paragraph is an appropriate time in which to incorporate suitable suggestions for your client should you choose to do so.

A 'standard' end-of-therapy routine

Use an appropriate induction and then proceed as follows:

> *"We have shared a great deal together to bring you to this wonderful moment of success and achievement. Today is a very special day because now it is time for you to move forward in your life with new awareness and understanding. You will find yourself taking more and more pride and great pleasure in how well you control your mind, your body and your emotions.*

> *"You will feel a warm golden glow of well-being deep within you and every day that warm, golden glow of well-being will grow. More today than yesterday but not nearly as much as it will tomorrow. Each day and every day finds you taking more and more control of your life as you become more confident about every aspect of your life.*

> *"Every day you will feel the benefit of your therapy and you will find the memory of me gradually fading away. Other people may notice the new self-assured, positive you, before you do. Well, that's okay, because each day and every day and for the rest of your days in some way you are going to improve something about yourself.*

"This calm confidence and self-assurance, this poised manner just builds up inside every day. It has always been there and it is going to persist inside you and it's going to remain and stay with you...

"You are going to become steadily more aware that so many of the things that could previously upset you, now just leave you feeling calm and relaxed when you deal with those things... dealing with them in a calm, relaxed, confident sort of way. You recognise and gratefully accept that you are your own master, at least the equal of any other and no one controls you... any more...

"Each day that goes by finds you thinking less and less about me and any feelings which you may have for me become less and less important as each day goes by. And you'll find yourself thinking more and more about really living, where previously you may have just been merely existing."

Part Four

Tidying Up

Chapter 26

Putting Things to Rights in the Client's Mind

There is a need in therapy that justice has at least to be seen to be done within the client's belief system. All too often clients will report that: "It's all very well but the bastard has got away with it". There is, though, a simple and effective way to facilitate a feeling of justice within the client's belief system.

We will begin by explaining why there is a necessity for a sense of justice to occur in the client's mind and not elsewhere. Imagine that you are restoring a car, a collector's car that you have been working on for twelve years. You have invested a lot of effort, spent every available spare hour and any spare cash on buying bits and pieces for your car. You keep your car in the garage and travel miles to find parts—in addition to all of this, you have joined several enthusiasts' clubs and your social life evolves around these to the exclusion of all else. It is simply a wonderful hobby, one of the most important things in your life.

One day you arrive home from work and you notice that the police are at your home, the front door is wide open, and neighbours come running out to meet you. The story begins to unfold. It appears two youths were seen in the neighbourhood—one tall and slim with ginger hair the other short stocky with dark hair and a scar on his upper lip. Noise was heard from your house, the garage door was opened and your car had been seen disappearing down the road with two people in it.

The police ask for a full description of the car, then tell you that the interior of your home has been totally wrecked. It does not stop there, though: the intruders have destroyed your pet hamsters and budgies, the bedroom walls have been smeared with excrement, all items of any value have been taken and everything that they could not carry has been wrecked almost beyond recognition.

Shock, horror, anger, disgust, revenge must all be going through your mind, so much so that the idea of sleeping in the house would be impossible to contemplate. And then you discover that there's urine and excrement in the bed. Could you ever sleep in that bed again?

The neighbours all show support and voice their opinions of the intruders, saying words like: "If I could get my hands on them I would skin them alive." Perhaps their words are echoing your thoughts. The police ask you to list everything that you can see is missing. Then they leave, after telling you that they will be in touch as soon they have some information.

You begin the process of rebuilding your home, a task that is a constant reminder of what has happened. Quite apart from the cost and/or wrangling with the insurance company, so much time is taken up looking for replacement items—those things that can be replaced, anyway. Some things are, quite simply, irreplaceable.

The probability is that, from this day forward, you will notice any collector's car that resembles yours, looking to see if there are two people in the car. Jewellers' shops that you walk past will always catch your eye as you look to see if by any chance something of yours is in the window. You would probably notice anybody and everybody who resembles your suspects, and perhaps would spend some considerable time studying the newspapers to see if any other similar robberies have been reported. It could even be that you would feel a temporary sense of justice if there were a report on the radio that a ginger-haired man was apprehended for something illegal.

A while after the robbery a policeman comes to your door and informs you that two youths have been sentenced, but, unfortunately, none of your possessions was found. The car had been vandalised and then set on fire. The officer looks on his list and says that they both got nine years each, after five other offences had been taken into consideration.

Now, how do you feel at that moment? Are you satisfied with the sentence? What if it had been more—say twenty years? Would that bring justice about? Let us assume that the sentence that you had in mind was, indeed, nine years.

Life now returns to a new normality. You are probably not likely to be continually looking for those two characters, nor looking out for a car that resembles yours. Your sleep is most likely to resume to normal. You would have a sense that justice had been done and you could now 'move on'.

Five years later you are happily walking along the road when a policeman whom you recognise from the time of the robbery stops you and says that he tried to contact you after the last visit because he had made an error. Where he had looked on his clipboard for the sentence he had looked in the wrong column and given the wrong sentence. It was in fact two years each, suspended for five years.

So what is this showing us? All that time that you believed that they were being punished, all was well. Our minds seek justice at being hurt; it is a very personal justice we seek, not society's justice. It needs to happen in our mind—it was our mind that gave us a feeling of justice having been done during the five years that we thought they were being punished. What if that police officer had not bumped into us? We would never have known of the error and would be none the wiser. What if he said that the reason that they were never found was that on the day of the robbery, they lost control of the car and crashed, both dying when it had rolled down a disused quarry and exploded in flames?

Ponder on the following: What if they are apprehended five years later? Would you still want justice? The law certainly demands it. What if that person says something like: "Oh come on, that was five years ago. I haven't done anything now, have I?" Well, he has a point. Right now he has not done anything wrong.

You may be wondering what this might have to do with therapy. In the mind justice must be done to make recompense for the injustice that was done to it, no matter how far back the injustice.

The courtroom of the mind

The client should imagine a courthouse, a grand structure, sturdy, solid and attractive-looking with the following elements:

- pillars that support the entrance

- bright lighting

- marble floor leading into the courtroom

- area for the accused

- area for the witnesses

- area for the victims

- area for reporters

- area for the public

- podium with judge's chair

- large video screen

The client is invited to either sit in judgement or to appoint a judge who has the wisdom and insight to deal with the accused in the most appropriate way.

Do not proceed any further with this technique unless all relevant material has been extracted during analytical therapy.

Now proceed as follows:

> *"Now slowly make your way towards the courthouse of your mind. See this beautiful grand structure and the marble steps that lead up to the main entrance. Inside you are pleased to note the quality of the fittings. Everything in its place and a place for everything. Doors open only when you will them to open. And as you approach the courtroom, the large solid doors part for you to enter. Inside there are areas for the victims, the accused, witnesses, etc. Make yourself comfortable in either the judge's chair, or a chair that allows you to see all that is happening in the courtroom. Let the victim/ victims enter the courtroom and see them all sitting. And I don't know what their ages are but you will see them all there in front of you. Now it is time for the accused to enter the courtroom."*

(This obviously may become fairly emotional for the client.)

The evidence has been submitted already and it is time for the judge to pass judgement. Help your client decide what sentence should be passed. The judge should give a sentence to the accused that is in direct relation to the feeling experienced by the victim. So if the child experienced unfairness the sentence will be unfair. If the child felt bullied then the judge will order that the accused be bullied until he has understood what it feels like to be bullied.

The judge has to ensure that whatever feelings—both physical and emotional—were created by the accused, must be returned to the accused. In some ways it is giving something back that was given to the client. In some instances this can become quite traumatic where the abuse was of a sexual nature. It is not always necessary to create a full-blown repeat of the incident as it is only designed to give back to the client's abuser the feeling of abuse.

In some cases the client has instructed that justice must take the form of sexual abuse where the abuser has himself to experience abuse of a sexual nature and the violation experienced by the client. This can be achieved by the client ordering the abuse of the abuser by a ten-foot monster so that the abuser would understand also how it feels to be powerless with someone twice your size.

The principal benefit of using the courtroom is that the client by the sheer fact of having the abusers in court has accepted that injustice was caused by the persons in the dock. The result is a sense of instant justice.

Other possible outcomes

It is quite possible that your client will suddenly feel sorry for the accused person and under these circumstances you will need to tread carefully. It may be that there has been a sudden understanding and forgiveness, or a feeling that by allowing punishment, he will descend to the level of the accused individual. Sometimes there may be a sudden sense of indifference about whatever has happened or a wish to somehow rise above it.

Whatever the reasons, whatever is being said, whatever the outcome in this courtroom of your client's mind, it is essential that he is content and convinced that either justice has been done, or that he has truly let go of the hurt.

Part Five

Miscellaneous

Chapter 27

The Reality of Abortion

This story is presented in this format so that the therapist may have some idea of the realities of abortion, allowing her to deal sensitively and knowledgeably with what is most definitely a traumatising situation.

I just knew, and it was strange, because I don't know how I knew. I had seen this guy in the local pubs quite a few times. He was like part of the group and gradually we just got chatting. Neither of us had partners. In fact I had been on my own for a long time. We were both very drunk and holding on to each other singing the songs from the disco.

It got to closing time and he invited me back to his place for a coffee. I knew he meant more than a coffee but by this time I didn't really care much. I just wanted to be with someone. We went to his place and I remember I was on the bed, he was undressing me, he was on top of me, I felt motionless.

Suddenly somewhere in my mind I was sober. All I kept thinking was "No condom—oh, Christ! No condom, I'm not on the pill!" It wasn't the thought of disease so much as the thought of being pregnant. I managed to get off the bed and stagger to the toilet and sat there for what seemed like ages thinking that maybe it would trickle out of me. I rested my head against the wall as I sat there reminding myself that I can't have children; I'm 32 and it's never happened yet, it's just not possible, I can't have children. Then I noticed the shower—one of those that's on a flex. Maybe I can wash it out. I want to wash anyway. So I did. Then I went downstairs. That drunk, sick feeling returned to my stomach and everything in my head was spinning. Eventually I fell asleep on the sofa.

In the morning he took me home and said "See yer". I knew he wouldn't.

For the next few weeks, I guess I shut it out. I felt really good, healthy, almost blossoming—in fact the best I'd felt in years, until I missed my period. Then I remembered. I got a pregnancy test kit, you know one of those you do at home and it proved positive. I just stood there in the bathroom looking at it in disbelief... the little capsule said I WAS PREGNANT. I sat on the side of the bath totally bewildered. I kept shaking the capsule like it was a thermometer or something but it didn't change.

That evening I went to the doctor, national health, I didn't have the money for private treatment. My doctor is a lovely lady and she tried very hard to talk me out of an abortion. "Think of your age my dear, your body clock is ticking away fast," she said. "Many women manage to bring a child up on their own."

"Not me!" I thought. "Just get me in the hospital and get this over with."

I had made my decision. The doctor contacted the local hospital there and then and I heard her say she had someone for a TOP. She gave me a form to fill in to take with me for my appointment the following week. In the next few days I didn't talk much to anyone. I made my excuses to my parents and went off to the hospital. The questioning I went through was the most degrading experience. "You're old enough to know better," was the doctor's closing comment.

The examination was vile. The nurse placed a condom over a sort of vibrator which was linked to a TV screen. The doctor inserts this thing into me and there on the screen was my insides.

"Yes, yes, there it is, I can see it," says the nurse and we all stare at the screen. There is my baby.

"OK, get dressed, Miss Lucas, and nurse will make an appointment for you for next Monday. Will someone be with you when you come in?"

"No."

The doctor turns to the nurse and says: "She'll have to stay overnight—arrange a bed."

I drive myself to the hospital.

As I walk into the ward I can't believe my eyes, they're all pregnant, how insensitive can these people be? Maybe it's part of the punishment because that's how they make you feel. Like you've done something wrong. I am taken into a side-room which has windows into the ward, the nurse closes the curtains and tells me to bath and put on the green gown that's on the bed, then she will come back. She returns with a white cup of liquid.

"This will stop the sickness after the anaesthetic, drink it all down," she says. I drank.

It wasn't long before I started to feel a bit woozy so I sat on the bed. Then came the injection and everything just seemed to fade away.

I could hear someone calling my name and as I opened my eyes I could see lots of lights and people in masks and tissue-type hats. For a moment I thought it was over but I'm having another injection. Someone is telling me to count backwards from one hundred. What comes after one hundred? I start to say some numbers, then nothingness.

The next time I open my eyes I have the most excruciating pain in my stomach. I cry out for some painkillers or something and two nurses come rushing over. One holds me up and one is holding a bowl to my chin. "Do you want to be sick, be sick here in the bowl."

"Give me something for the pain!" I'm screaming at her by this time.

"No, no, you'll be fine, come on, be a good girl and be sick now." I want to tell her to fuck off and just get me something for the pain. Maybe this is how they punish you.

They take me back to the room and give me something to make me sleep.

At about 6 in the evening a woman comes in, wakes me up and offers me some food. I don't want anything, so she leaves. I sit up to get a drink of water and on the bedside cabinet is a sanitary towel the size of a pillow. I notice I'm wearing a white gown now. I lift the covers to see if it goes all the way down and there is blood everywhere. I panic inside, I feel hot and get this rushing sensation in my head. I ring the buzzer and a nurse comes in.

"Oh, you're all right, put this sanitary towel on and get into your own night clothes," she says, then gets a clean sheet for the bed and takes away the blood-stained gown. I fall asleep.

It's about 2 in the morning when I wake up. I want a cigarette and I remember there is a coffee machine at the end of the corridor by the visitors' room. I put my cigarettes in my dressing-gown pocket and very slowly walk to the machine and get a coffee. I notice another woman in the visitors' room. We just smile. As I take out a cigarette she asks if she can have one and the conversation begins. She tells me that her baby died inside her and she had to have it removed. She has been trying for years to have a child. She starts to cry. I put my arms around her and I'm thinking: "Please don't ask me why I'm here." As I'm thinking it, she asks.

"My baby died, too," I said.

The woman continued to cry while I held her. I felt nothing for myself. In the morning, as I left, the nurse gave me some antibiotics and told me if I continue bleeding after a week to go to my doctor. I walked to the car, threw my bag in the boot and started to drive home. It was a very sunny day, springtime. I turned on the radio and heard the Supremes—"Baby love, my baby love, I need you, oh how I need you."

I started to feel all this emotion inside, in my chest and my eyes began to fill with tears. It seemed as if I turned off the radio and pulled the car over all at the same time. I began to cry.

Oh God, what have I done?

There is often a lack of information available to assist us when working with clients who have been through the experience of an abortion. The following is based purely on work carried out in the consulting room and it will almost certainly be of help to you and your clients.

The most powerful emotion at work here is guilt. The woman will frequently talk to us about her abortion in a very matter-of-fact way initially, using phrases like:

"Just one of those things."

"Well, it wasn't life yet."

"I've dealt with it now, I'm fine."

Some women have an abortion because:

"It was a mistake."

"I/we already have enough children."

In cases of this kind there may be anger towards the partner mixed with guilt; the anger will need to be released and the guilt worked through. Some women feel pushed by their partner into having an abortion, especially where there has been manipulation along the lines of: "If you have this baby, I'm leaving."

Here, you can expect feelings of fear and rejection to play a major part in any symptom formation and this client will need to release all the associated repressed, or suppressed, feelings before you apply your confidence—and ego-boosting skills.

Some other thoughts

Very young girls who have had abortions will often have been encouraged to do so by a parent or guardian.

In cases where the abortion is a secret, your client will feel some relief just by telling you about it.

The abortion can most definitely have had an effect on the father— so do not dismiss this with your male clients. The emotional response can be remarkably similar to that of women and can include anger and hatred towards the partner.

Some of your clients will have been offered counselling by the hospital, so it is always a good idea to ask if this has occurred. Was she offered any form of assistance at that time? Did she find it helpful? Quite frequently, your client will have been referred to a family planning clinic which does not always offer counselling but rather pills and condoms, coils and caps, etc—and, in some instances, a lecture.

The women who have had to have their pregnancy aborted because the baby was found to be damaged or unhealthy in some way often *will* show some emotion. In most of these cases you would use a script about how nature knows best. This can also be used in cases of miscarriage.

It is rare indeed for a client to present with symptoms that she believes to be the after-effects of an abortion. Where it is reported that this has happened, though, it is almost inevitable that it will be at least *partly* responsible for whatever symptom pattern exists.

Symptoms of an abortion

Some common symptoms of abortion are:

- the client may hold her current partner responsible

- the client may punish her children

- the client may never have children

- the client may find a partner who cannot have children

Where there is any unusual attitude towards children or the procreative process, always check as thoroughly as you sensitively can, to ascertain whether or not there has been an abortion or 'procured miscarriage'.

Chapter 28

Some Symptoms of Psychosis

Every therapist should be aware of the Golden Rule of *Neurotics not Psychotics* being taken into analytical therapy. In practice, though, it is sometimes quite difficult to be certain exactly where that dividing line between neurosis and psychosis actually is, and some psychotically ill individuals can be very deceptive, often appearing to be quite intelligent and even superficially charming. It is as wrong to assume that you can recognise an individual with this illness by his appearance or demeanour, as it is to believe that he is always dangerous.

When you have little or no experience of mental illness, it is very easy to hold a belief that you would always be able to tell if someone was 'mad', mainly because most people have quite a few inaccurate ideas about what 'madness', or psychosis, actually is. It is nothing to do with intelligence levels, though many psychotics will actually have an IQ far higher than the average person. They do not have 'mad eyes' or *necessarily* a strange or awkward manner—in fact, they can be extraordinarily charming and super-ficially very successful. These are the ones you are most likely to meet in your consulting room from time to time.

But they can also be withdrawn and isolated; unwashed, unkempt and totally passive; gesticulating wildly and talking to themselves; standing on street corners, staring at nothing in particular; rummaging around in litter bins; indulging in strange rituals that make no sense to anybody but themselves (and may be mistaken as merely an obsessive personality); they might have bizarre clothes or hairstyles or they may dress in a uniform that has absolutely nothing whatsoever to do with them at all—RAF, police, doctor, Commando, etc.; they might make very convincing claims of persecution… the list could go on, but you get the idea.

The one thing that is certain about schizophrenia is that it is totally devastating and the most severe of mental illnesses. As it progresses, there is a gradual deterioration in an individual's work until he simply cannot go to work, along with increasing difficulties with social relationships and in caring for himself. This can happen so insidiously that immediate friends and family of the sufferer may not realise there is anything actually wrong at all until the illness is fairly well advanced, and even then there is usually an unwillingness to accept reality, maybe with claims that "He's just a bit difficult to understand sometimes, that's all."

Where behaviour and speech patterns are noticeably 'odd'—there are sometimes disturbances in the motor system, like rigidity, with a posture being held for ages, or, more commonly, what looks like excessive animation which soon shows itself to be without purpose and oddly repetitive—this sometimes causes others to laugh, maybe even believing that the unfortunate sufferer is indulging in some kind of jokey behaviour. The sufferer may even seem to go along with this to an extent, though he is really on a totally different wavelength and his behaviour patterns are rooted in frustration and desperation, rather than a sense of fun. His emotional responses will sometimes seem flat, sometimes inappropriate in some other way.

The term *schizophrenia*—probably the most common form of psychosis—actually refers to not one, but a group of psychotic illnesses which often start in adolescence or young adulthood. There tend to be 'attacks' with gaps in between, typically starting at about 15 years old. Between attacks the sufferer can seem quite normal, though the frequency of attacks will tend to increase— slowly if the environment is good (stable home, low excitation levels, low 'life-difficulties', supportive relatives, etc.) but faster if not (homelessness, frustration, angry/nagging relatives or companions, stress of any sort). The symptoms are varied and include severe and obvious disturbances in perception, emotion and thought; difficulties in sustaining 'normal' relationships with others; an odd or unrealistic sense of self; detachment from reality; and gradually diminishing abilities to communicate or even function at a social level. The lay expression 'split personality' that is often used to describe this group of illnesses is inaccurate, since it really describes MPD (Multiple Personality Disorder), which is a very different kettle of fish indeed. The word *schizophrenia* was coined in 1911 by a Swiss psychiatrist called Eugen Bleuler to replace Emile Kraepelin's *dementia praecox*, and it means 'shattered mind' and refers, in fact, to the dissociation between the emotions and cognition, between reality and delusion.

There is a distinct difficulty in separating reality from imagination and dreams. Fantasy often plays a large part in the schizophrenic's life and can be very vivid and, to him, apparently totally real. I say apparently, because he seems to believe his tales completely and it is impossible to tell whether this is the case or if he is just sticking to the story he's invented. Certainly those stories will be told consistently and it can be difficult to find flaws in them. There is little doubt that, to the schizophrenic, the tales he tells *are* real.

There can be an inherited predisposition with some individuals—the disorder definitely runs in families. Children who have one schizophrenic parent have *ten times* the chance of developing the disorder than if their parent had been 'normal'. During your information gathering, you should always enquire as to the emotional and psychological health of your client's parents. If he tells you that one of them was excessively *anything* that could be taken to indicate schizophrenia, then explore your client's psyche that much more carefully.

Sufferers used to be kept in asylums for long periods, if not the whole of their life; more often, now, they are treated with the latest genre of powerful tranquillisers and are able to lead a normal life, as long as they keep on taking their medication. Unfortunately, they often tend to have difficulty in accepting that there is anything actually wrong with them at all and for this reason do not always maintain the medication regime without constant supervision. It is no exaggeration to say that they usually believe that their ideas, however odd, are normal—and that it is the rest of the world that is out of step with *them.*

The advice to the GP about diagnosing schizophrenia is that any one of the symptoms from the first group, below, or two from the second group should have been present most of the time for a period of no less than one month:

Group One
Thought echo, withdrawal, insertion or broadcasting
Delusions of control or passivity
Delusional perception
Third person hallucinatory voices
Persistent bizarre delusions

Group Two
Persistent hallucinations in any modality.
Thought blocking and disorder
Neologisms
Catatonia
Apathy, poverty of speech or thought
Blunting of effect and social withdrawal

Many of the symptoms on those lists are self-explanatory, though some may need clarifying.

Thought Echo is a type of hallucination in which the sufferer hears his thoughts being spoken aloud, as if by a third party.

Thought broadcasting is that state where the thoughts are experienced as being broadcast aloud from one's head, so loud that they can easily be heard by others.

Thought insertion refers to the belief of the sufferer that 'someone' has forced a thought repeatedly into his mind.

Thought withdrawal is an experience that, somehow or another, one's thoughts have been taken away. Sometimes there is an accompanying feeling that there are fewer thoughts left to use.

Delusions of control can mean that the sufferer truly believes he can cause global or universal effects at will—one of the forms of delusions of grandeur. This is not unlike the so-called 'magical thinking' of children up to the age of 8 or so, where the child believes that his thoughts can directly affect his environment and will make vigorous attempts to exercise this skill against enemies (which may include parents and/or siblings). Much of the behaviour of schizophrenics, in fact, seems to echo that of children, when you examine it closely.

The French playwright Rostand ably illustrated delusions of control in one of his works thus: "I recoil, overcome with the glory of my rosy hue and the knowledge that I, a mere cock, have made the sun rise." It can also mean that there is the belief that someone, somewhere, is in control of the sufferer—he will seriously inform you that some device has been inserted into his brain during a medical operation or a period of forceful restraint by police or some other authority and who now controls him.

Delusional perception includes delusions of grandeur and claims of persecution and/or harassment from gangs/groups/doctors/police etc. Often these delusions are gross distortions of normal events, so that a train strike would be considered proof that 'they' are trying to stop him from getting away.

Persistent bizarre delusions include claims to be in a position of power—a Captain in the SAS, for example—or authority, or maybe an insistence that he has a special secret mission to perform. There can be assertions of approaching catastrophe that only he knows about, often to do with Russians or space aliens, or perhaps extreme role-playing that may even extend to wearing costume, acting the part well enough to fool most people and believing it fully himself—doctors, nurses, firemen, policemen are commonly adopted roles.

Neologisms are words or phrases that make no real sense, even though they might at first appear to. Sometimes, they can take the form of a 'title', or a career or vocation which will sound plausible and 'special', but has no connection with reality and no basis in fact. There will sometimes be a degree of grandiosity.

The 1992 classification of schizophrenia lists five types: paranoid, hebephrenic, catatonic, residual and simple.

Paranoid schizophrenia is the most commonly recognised form, with delusions of persecution, threatening hallucinatory voices and fear among the more noticeable symptoms. Within true paranoia, the individual insists that he is an extremely important person, or holds an extremely important position, and that others (which may include people like the Queen, the police, or simply a huge gang of thugs) are determined to 'get' him.

Hebephrenic schizophrenia symptoms include brief hallucinations and delusions, thought disorder and odd or affected mannerisms and/or behaviour patterns which may include walking with a strange gait, behaving in a 'camp' manner, or laughing hysterically at some repeated action which is not at all funny to the onlooker. There may also be 'silly' affectations of speech, pronouncing words in an unusual manner, etc.

In **catatonic schizophrenia** motor disturbances are prominent and may include stupor, non-responsiveness, sudden bouts of excitement or hyperkinesis (pathologically increased muscle movement—whole body tic), and preservation of posture ('freezing'—maybe for hours at a time, or until the limbs are actually rearranged by someone else). This is a very rare form of the illness.

Residual schizophrenia is a chronic stage which often follows the three previously mentioned and is dominated by withdrawal, isolation, apathy, and blunted emotional response. It looks like severe depression and is marked by a total apparent lack of awareness of others.

Simple schizophrenia is an uncommon disorder with a continual but slow development of unusual behaviour and social decline. Vagrancy and homelessness may result. The sufferer may not wash for months or years, nor groom himself in any way at all. Those sad individuals you can sometimes see pushing supermarket trolleys full of junk fall into this category.

There are around 10,000 new cases of schizophrenia diagnosed every year; the risk of developing it during the course of a lifetime is reported to be in the region of 1 in 100. In its full form it is very obvious and you should be easily able to spot it during your initial consultation—though it has to be said that you will get few 'full-blooded' schizophrenia sufferers coming to you. But there is a borderline 'grey' area into which many neurotics fit just as easily as *potential* psychotics, and this is where we have to be careful.

Presenting symptoms to be wary of include:

(1)   Temper outbursts that are uncontrollable and invariably lead to violence, especially where there appears to be no great concern about this—this client will often have presented himself for something quite different and may view his outbursts with amusement.

(2)   Symptoms that do not quite make sense—one young man stated seriously that: "I never seem to know what my eyes are saying. And I often realise that I'm not in my own time." Insects or other foreign organisms/materials inhabiting the physiology, sometimes reportedly left there by surgeons or aliens, obviously come into this category.

(3)   An intense dislike of mixing with 'the average person'.

(4)   Intense dislike or hatred of several members of the immediate family.

(5)   An intense dislike of hearing other people eat/talk/shout/laugh, etc.

(6)   An inability to feel comfortable with people at all—often preferring animals.

(7)   An excessive anxiety about any authority figure.

(8)   A constant feeling of being in danger—often after some event or occasion where the sufferer was, either in reality or fantasy, pursued by others for no apparent reason.

(9)   A belief that most people are 'out to get' anybody who drops his guard.

(10) Profound anxiety/panic arising from some extreme event, either real or imaginary.

(11) 'Tall' stories about success/failure/prowess, etc.

(12) An excessive repugnance of other people's normal bodily functions, leading to extreme anger or a wish to harm/punish others.

If you find either of the first two above, or three or more of the others along with a behaviour pattern or way of being that seems in any way 'odd' or unusual, then you should be extremely cautious about taking this would-be client into therapy. When an individual seems not to fit into that broad band of what we call 'normal', even if you cannot define why it seems like that to you, then ask a lot of questions based around the above twelve points, wanting 'normal' answers and responses before agreeing to work with him. Where there is any doubt in your mind, trust your gut reaction and *never* go against it, preferring to err on the side of caution rather than risk making someone more ill than he was to start off with—and rather than find yourself having to deal with someone who is *mentally* ill (as opposed to *emotionally* ill) and maybe way outside your 'area of expertise'. Those doubts would be likely to preclude a successful analysis, anyway.

This bears repetition because it is so important: you *simply cannot tell* whether or not an individual is schizophrenic from the appearance alone. The psychotic often has a very high IQ and will not infrequently be a 'high-flier' of some sort in commerce or industry, or maybe running—or claiming to run—a hugely successful business or two. That, in itself, veers away from the norm and should prompt you to find out more. Obviously, not all successful people are psychotic, nor are all psychotic people successful, but the circumstance of a genuinely intelligent, successful, smartly presented and superficially charming psychotic is far from unknown.

It can be quite difficult to say 'no', but you will have to do it on occasions. You can say something along the lines of: "Well, (name), it certainly seems that you do need some help, but I don't feel that hypnosis is the best therapy for you. I think you should go to your GP and tell him your symptoms, just as you've explained them to me, and ask his advice." This usually does the trick, but if he won't budge in his belief that hypnosis *is* the answer, the best response is probably along the lines of: "Well, you *may* be right, and of course you can always seek a second opinion." It doesn't matter a great deal what you say, as long as you are polite but firm and get him out of your consulting room.

You should always try to leave anybody that you refuse therapy to with a positive idea of where he *can* seek treatment. He has come to you for help and the fact that you cannot be of assistance to him is not his fault, whatever the reason, so you should attempt to avoid leaving him with a sense of hopelessness. Our duty of care is to everyone who comes into our consulting room seeking our help, not just to those whom we take on as clients.

A LAST WORD

In all of the forms of hypnotherapy and psychotherapy, there really is no 'best method', only methods that work best for any particular client. Whilst the authors of this book would not claim that what is presented here is in any way a panacea for all emotional ills, it *is* fair to say that there are very few situations indeed that can arise in the consulting chair for which you could not at least find something here which will be of help.

As with all therapeutic endeavour, the ingenuity of the therapist and the relationship between the therapist and the client are of paramount importance—and there is plenty here to help you achieve excellence in both ingenuity and client-rapport building. We hope that you will take our offering, add your own self to it, and turn it into something truly spectacular!

Goodbye for the moment ... and good luck.

Georges Philips and Terence Watts

For details of workshops, seminars and training please contact Georges Philips on 020 8446 2210 or via www.icet.net

References

pg. 9   Michael D. Yapko *Trancework*—Michael Yapko is a clinical psychologist in San Diego as well as director of the Milton H. Erikson Institute of San Diego—Published by Brunner/Mazel, 19 Union Square West, New York, NY 1003

pg. 61   'The work of Dave Elman' Dave Elman *Hypnotherapy* Published by Westwood Publishing Co.

pg. 72   The Watkins Affect Bridge technique 'The Affect Bridge' *International Journal of Clinical and Experimental Hypnosis*, 1971, 19, 28.

pg. 90   David Grove's 'Effective reflective language'. The subject of a lecture by the English psychotherapist, author David Grove

pg. 147   Table-top therapy™ —Georges Philips and Lyn Buncher 1994

pg. 198   'Adapted from a technique by Milton Erickson' *My Voice Will Go With You* Edited by Sidney Rosen—Published by London W W Norton & Company

pg. 200   'Based around work by E. A. Barnet, MD' *Analytical Hypnotherapy* E. A. Barnet, MD. Published by Westwood Publishing Co.

pg. 235   Quote from Rostand—source unknown.

Bibliography

Andreas, C., & Andreas, S., (1989) *Heart of the Mind*, Moab, Utah: Real People Press.

Andreas, S., & Andreas, C., (1987) *Change Your Mind and Keep the Change*, Moab, Utah: Real People Press.

Andreas, S., & Faulkner, C., (1994) *NLP: The New Technology of Achievement*, London: Brealey Publishing.

Bandler, R., (1985) *Using Your Brain for a Change*, Moab, Utah: Real People Press.

Bandler, R., & Grinder, J., (1975) *Frogs into Princes*, Moab, Utah: Real People Press.

Bandler, R., & Grinder, J., (1975) *Patterns of the Hypnotic Techniques of Milton H. Erickson, M.D.*, Cupertino, California: Meta Publications.

Bandler, R., & Grinder, J., (1975) *Reframing: Neuro-Linguistic Programming and the Transformation of Meaning*, Moab, Utah: Real People Press.

Bandler, R., & Grinder, J., (1975) *The Structure of Magic Vol. I*, Palo Alto: Science & Behavior Books Inc.

Barnet, E.A., (1989) *Analytical Hypnotherapy Principles & Practice*, Glendale, California: Westwood Publishing.

Cameron-Bandler, L., Gordon, D., & Lebeau, M., (1985) *The Emprint Method: A Guide to Reproducing Competence*, Moab, Utah: Real People Press.

D. Corydon Hammond, Ph.D., edited by; (1990) *The Handbook of Hypnotic Suggestions and Metaphors,* London: W W Norton & Company.

Dilts, R., (1990) *Changing Belief Systems with NLP*, Capitola, California: Meta Publications.

Dilts, R., (1994) *Strategies of Genius, Vol 1.*, Capitola, California: Meta Publications.

Dilts, R., Grinder, J., Bandler, R., & DeLozier J., (1978) *Neuro-Linguistic Programming: The Study of the Structure of Subjective Experience, Vol I*, Cupertino, California: Meta Publications.

Elman, David, (1984) *Hypnotherapy,* Glendale, California:Westwood Publishing.

Grinder, J. & Bandler, R., (1981) *Trance-formations: Neuro-Linguistic Programming and the Structure of Hypnosis*, Moab, Utah: Real People Press.

Hall, E.T., (1959) *The Silent Language*, New York: Doubleday and Co Ltd.

Hunter, Roy C., (1995) *The Art of Hypnotherapy*, Dubuque: Kendal/Hunt Publishing Co.

Jacoby, Mario, (1995) *The Analytical Encounter*, Toronto: Inner City Books.

Jacobson, S., (1983) *Meta-cation*, Cupertino, California: Meta Publications.

Jung, C.G., (1969) *Jung Extracts: The Psychology of the Transference*, Boston, Massachusetts: Princeton University Press.

Lankton, S., (1980) *Practical Magic: A Translation of Basic Neuro-Linguistic programming into Clinical Psychotherapy*, Cupertino, California: Meta Publications.

Lewis, B., & Pucelik, F., (1990) *Magic of NLP Demystified: A Pragmatic Guide To Communication & Change*, Portland Oregon: Metamorphous Press.

Peiffer, Vera, (1996) *Principles of Hypnotherapy*, London: Thorsons.

Philips, George and Buncher, Lyn, (1999) *Gold Counselling® The Practical Psychology with NLP Second Edition,* Carmarthen: Crown House Publishing Ltd.

Rosen, Sidney, Ed. *My Voice Will Go With You*, London: W W Norton & Company

Sasz, Thomas, (1988) *The Ethics of Psychoanalysis*, Syracuse: Syracuse Univ. Press.

Michael D. Yapko (1990) *Trancework* Philadelphia: Brunner/Mazel Publishers.

Index

Ability 111, 153, 160, 185, 191-192
Abortion 225-230
Abreaction 26-27, 29, 82-84, 132
Abuse 78, 94-95, 114, 171, 197, 221
Accessing 5, 129, 131-133, 135
Accused 26, 220-221
Achilles 25, 27, 29
Addiction 24
Adolescence 232
Adult 7, 9, 11, 35, 37, 43-44, 114-116, 182, 203
Advice 92, 159, 200, 233, 238
After-effects 230
Age 81, 84, 104-105, 114, 131, 147, 226, 234
Aggression 37
Agoraphobia 6, 69, 82
Aliens 4, 6, 235, 237
Alleviate 87, 197
Ancestral 34, 185, 187, 189, 191-193, 195
Anchor 137, 185
Andreas, S. and Andreas, C. 243
Anger 26, 37, 42, 83, 201, 217, 229, 237
Angry 150-151, 190, 232
Anguish 24
Anorexics 9
Anorgasmia 71
Archetypes 185, 187, 189, 191, 193, 195
Arms 14, 29, 64-65, 84, 101, 156, 191, 197, 208, 228
Asleep 13, 225, 228
Assertiveness 37, 185
Associated 10, 32, 69, 95, 100-101, 132, 158, 185, 195, 198, 229
Attitude 26-27, 151, 188, 230
Auditory 84, 111
Awareness 20, 27, 36, 120, 152-153, 156, 173-174, 185, 212, 236

Baby 171, 226, 228-230
Bandler, R. 243
Barnet, E.A. 241, 243
Behavioural 137, 140
Behaviours 57
Beliefs 3, 7
Benefit 18, 37, 57, 107, 125, 212, 221
Benefits 50, 120
Bind 53, 56
Bio-feedback 14, 72, 79, 95
Black-outs 30, 71
Bleuler, Eugen 232
Blindness 30, 71
Blockages 126
Blocked 126-127
Blood 166, 210, 228

Bonding 197-198
Borderline 236
Bowel 24, 185
Brain 245, 62, 90, 198, 235
Breathing 64, 66, 156, 175, 207, 209, 211
Brief 23, 25, 27, 29, 31, 63, 70, 130, 236
Bullied 26, 131, 221
Bullying 8, 81
Buncher, Lyn 243, 244
Business 17, 71, 78, 98, 100, 112, 114, 186, 238,

Calm 26, 44, 90, 125, 151, 156, 182, 207, 213
Cameron-Bandler, Leslie 243
Care 8, 24, 171, 187, 225, 239
Caring 28, 32, 188, 232
Catalysts 20
Catatonic 235-236
Changework 22, 201-202
Charisma 30, 77, 191
Charismatic 24-25, 29, 32, 64, 188, 194
Childhood 7, 35, 41-44, 69, 71, 77, 79, 81, 176, 195, 203
Children 9, 11, 37, 43, 103, 116, 225, 229-230, 233-234
Chinese 190
Choice 138, 155-156, 168, 189, 192, 200
Christ 225
Claustrophobia 69, 82, 174
Client-rapport 240
Cognition 233
Comfort-level 129, 203
Communication 116, 119, 160
Conflict 25-27, 29, 56, 70, 95, 99, 104, 148-149, 187
Conflicts 9, 34, 69
Congruence 40
Consciousness 7, 84, 135
Conversation 23, 27-28, 176, 178, 183-184, 228
Counselling 230
Counsellor 149
Counter-suggestion 9
Crying 131, 179
Crystals 103

Deepener 63-64, 66, 72, 79, 111, 200
Defence-mechanisms 152
Defence-strategy 152
Deletions 91
Delozier, Judith 243
Delusions 234-236
Dementia 232
Dependence 24

GOLD Counselling® Second Edition
A Structured Psychotherapeutic Approach To The Mapping And Re-Aligning Of Belief Systems
Georges Philips & Lyn Buncher
with Brian Stevenson

This highly acclaimed work has now been completely revised and expanded to reflect the latest advances made in the field. This second edition is an extensive expansion upon the original work, providing a wealth of additional material on beliefs. Nearly all change work, be it in counselling, psychotherapy or change in a business setting, involx ves changing beliefs in some way or another. This book sets out to explain, in easily understandable terms, what beliefs are, how they are formulated in our mind, the impact they have on our identity, and, most important of all, how they can be changed successfully. It also provides many worked examples to demonstrate the strategies involved as an aid to learning.

PAPERBACK   320 PAGES   ISBN: 1899836330

"Amazing, GOLD Counselling has become my most preferred method of helping clients help themselves. It has made me more efficient, effective and more confident."
– *Lyne Driscoll, counsellor a nd therapist.*

"*GOLD Counselling* has helped me to understand and change parts of myself and my beliefs I have been struggling with for years in various other forms of therapy. I have already seen the beneficial effects this is having on my life and on the therapy I am able to offer others as a result."
– *Dr Anne Curtis, psychosexual therapist and psychotherapist.*

"A quantum leap in restructuring and reforming beliefs. *GOLD Counselling* is a great asset for all NLP practitioners."
– *Steve Peet, Certified Trainer of NLP and lecturer at the University of London.*

Analytical Hypnotherapy Volume 1
Theoretical Principles
Jacquelyne Morison
with contributions from Georges Philips

A groundbreaking reference for everyone in the fields of hypnotherapy, psychotherapy and counselling, this book contains a complete explication of the theory behind analytical hypnotherapy. An eclectic, wide-ranging book, *Analytical Hypnotherapy Volume 1* examines not only the orthodox analytical approach, but also aspects of humanistic thinking and cognitive strategies which concentrate on activating the client's unconscious mind. Presenting a unique investigation into the ways in which analytical hypnotherapy has influenced a range of current therapeutic philosophies, *Analytical Hypnotherapy Volume 1* presents the clinical practitioner with the ultimate means of treating even the most stubborn of therpeutic disorders.

HARDBACK   448 PAGES   ISBN: 1899836772

"I consider this book ESSENTIAL for anyone involved in hypnotherapy."
– *Vera Peiffer, hypnotherapist and author.*

"A remarkable book that I would unhesitatingly recommend to both students and seasoned practitioners alike ... a modern classic."
– *William Broom, Chief Executive and Registrar, The General Hypnotherapy Standards Council.*

"I believe that practitioners will be enriched by, and clients benefit from, the vast corpus of knowledge and wisdom contained within this comprehensively-researched and well-written book."
– *Anne Billings, Fellow of the National Association of Counsellors, Hypnotherapists and Psychotherapists.*

Analytical Hypnotherapy Volume 2
Practical Applications
Jacquelyne Morison
with contributions from Georges Philips

In this sequel to the highly acclaimed first volume, Jacquelyne Morison introduces the clinical practitioner to the practical applications of analytical hypnotherapy – the process of transforming theory into practice. Providing a succinct and all-embracing overview of the topic, the author not only removes the mystery enshrouding the practice, but also brings analytical hypnotherapy into the mainstream of clinical techniques. *Analytical Hypnotherapy Volume 2* allows the hypnotherapist to accomplish an in-depth examination of the client's psyche. Equally, psychotherapists and counsellors will benefit from this invaluable guide, which aptly demonstrates the importance of hypnotherapy in investigative methodology and practice.

HARDBACK   496 PAGES   ISBN: 1899836853

"This book should be all that a therapist, either studying or already practising hypnoanalysis, will ever need."
– *Pat Doohan, Fellow of the National Council of Psychotherapists.*

"An excellent, comprehensive text, and a creative tool for practitioners in successfully bridging that significant interface between theory and practice."
– *Colin Hunter, hypnotherapist and healer.*

"This book is a gold-mine of information, well-written, clearly set out, and easy to learn from. I predict that this book will be the bible for any hypnotherapist who wants to get to the top of their profession."
– *Vera Peiffer, hypnotherapist and author.*

USA & Canada orders to:
Crown House Publishing
P.O. Box 2223, Williston, VT 05495-2223, USA
Tel: 877-925-1213, Fax: 802-864-7626
E-mail: info@CHPUS.com
www.CHPUS.com

UK & Rest of World orders to:
The Anglo American Book Company Ltd.
Crown Buildings, Bancyfelin, Carmarthen, Wales SA33 5ND
Tel: +44 (0)1267 211880/211886, Fax: +44 (0)1267 211882
E-mail: books@anglo-american.co.uk
www.anglo-american.co.uk

Australasia orders to:
Footprint Books Pty Ltd.
Unit 4/92A Mona Vale Road, Mona Vale NSW 2103, Australia
Tel: +61 (0) 2 9997 3973, Fax: +61 (0) 2 9997 3185
E-mail: info@footprint.com.au
www.footprint.com.au

Singapore orders to:
Publishers Marketing Services Pte Ltd.
10-C Jalan Ampas #07-01
Ho Seng Lee Flatted Warehouse, Singapore 329513
Tel: +65 6256 5166, Fax: +65 6253 0008
E-mail: info@pms.com.sg
www.pms.com.sg

Malaysia orders to:
Publishers Marketing Services Pte Ltd
Unit 509, Block E, Phileo Damansara 1, Jalan 16/11
46350 Petaling Jaya, Selangor, Malaysia
Tel : 03 7955 3588, Fax : 03 7955 3017
E-mail: pmsmal@po.jaring.my
www.pms.com.sg

South Africa orders to:
Everybody's Books
PO Box 201321, Durban North, 4016, RSA
Tel: +27 (0) 31 569 2229, Fax: +27 (0) 31 569 2234
E-mail: warren@ebbooks.co.za